The Power of Belief

Psychosocial Influence on Illness, Disability and Medicine

The Power of Belief
Psychosocial Influence on Illness, Disability and Medicine

Edited by

Peter W. Halligan
School of Psychology, Cardiff University, Cardiff, UK
and

Mansel Aylward
UnumProvident Centre for Psychosocial and Disability
Research, School of Psychology, Cardiff University,
Cardiff, UK

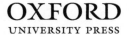

OXFORD
UNIVERSITY PRESS

This book has been printed digitally and produced in a standard specification
in order to ensure its continuing availability

OXFORD
UNIVERSITY PRESS

Great Clarendon Street, Oxford OX2 6DP

Oxford University Press is a department of the University of Oxford.
It furthers the University's objective of excellence in research, scholarship,
and education by publishing worldwide in

Oxford New York

Auckland   Cape Town Dar es Salaam   Hong Kong   Karachi
Kuala Lumpur Madrid Melbourne Mexico City   Nairobi
New Delhi Shanghai Taipei Toronto
With offices in
Argentina Austria Brazil Chile Czech Republic France Greece
Guatemala Hungary Italy Japan South Korea Poland Portugal
Singapore Switzerland Thailand Turkey Ukraine Vietnam

ISBN 978-0-19-853010-7

Acknowledgements

The editors would like to acknowledge the generous support provided by The Royal Society of Medicine in co-sponsoring and organising with the School of Psychology and the Department of Work and Pensions (Cardiff University) the conference, May 2003 that inspired this book.

We would like to thank Sue Dentten, Tracy Straker, Louise Morris, Lorriane Woods and Laura Morris for their assistance, in facilitating the conference and the subsequent book. Finally, we would also like to thank the staff at Oxford University Press.

Contents

List of Contributors

Mansel Aylward
UnumProvident Centre for
Psychosocial and Disability Research,
School of Psychology,
Cardiff University,
Cardiff, UK

Vaughan Bell
School of Psychology,
Cardiff University,
Cardiff, UK

Rachelle Buchbinder
Department of Clinical
Epidemiology, Cabrini Hospital,
Melbourne, Victoria, Australia

A. Kim Burton
Centre for Health and
Social Care Research,
University of Huddersfield, UK

Quinton Deeley
Institute of Psychiatry,
London, UK

Duncan B. Double
School of Medicine,
Health Policy and Practice,
University of East Anglia,
Norwich, UK

Hadyn D. Ellis
School of Psychology,
Cardiff University, Cardiff, UK

Robert Ferrari
University of Alberta Hospital,
Edmonton, AL, Canada

Jon Friel
Edmonton, AL, Canada

Kathleen M. Griffiths
Centre for Mental Health
Research, Australian
National University,
Canberra ACT, Australia

Peter W. Halligan
School of Psychology,
Cardiff University,
Cardiff, UK

Rob Horne
Centre for Health Care
Research, University of
Brighton, UK

Anthony F. Jorm
ORYGEN Research Centre,
University of Melbourne,
Melbourne Victoria,
Australia

Irving Kirsch
Department of Psychology,
University of Plymouth, UK

Oliver Kwan
Edmonton AL, Canada

Chris J. Main
Unit for Chronic Disease
Epidemiology,
University of Manchester, UK

David F. Marks
Department of Psychology,
City University,
London, UK

Peter Salmon
Department of Clinical Psychology,
University of Liverpool, UK

Gordon Waddell
Centre for Psychosocial and
Disability Research,
University of Cardiff, UK

Derick T. Wade
Oxford Centre for Enablement,
Oxford, UK

Beliefs: shaping experience and understanding illness

Peter W. Halligan

Man is what he believes.
Anton Chekhov

Some things have to be believed to be seen.
Ralph Hodgson

In every aspect of life, be it business, politics, religion, relationships, academia or healthcare, we make judgments, form interpretations and come to conclusions largely based on pre-existing notions about ourselves, our friends and the nature of reality. These pre-existing notions or beliefs (Lazarus and Folkman, 1984) are conceptually different from other sources of knowledge in that they involve a personal acceptance and often a public endorsement of a proposition or state of affairs that we hold to be evidently true and beyond empirical enquiry. This everyday or folk understanding of the nature and function of belief predates recent psychological explanations (see Gilbert, 1993) and provides for the existence of 'many non-scientific social institutions that are deeply entrenched in our culture, not least of which are the governmental system, the legal system, the educational system and the social service systems' (Green, 1995).

Although discussion of beliefs can be found in most health psychology (Janz & Becker, 1984; Ogden, 2004) and biopsychosocial models (White, 2005), the meaning of the term is typically assumed and used descriptively as one of several 'psychosocial variables' that impact on health and illness outcome.

Despite growing acceptance of biopsychosocial factors over the past three decades, comparatively few adopt the approach in clinical practice (Gilbert, 2002) and the evidence-based research, while promising, is still relatively small. One reason for this is that traditional biopsychosocial approaches are under-specified and poorly understood (Gilbert, 1995; Kiesler, 1999). Since Engel's seminal paper in 1977, (White, 2005) the biopsychosocial model has evolved. Over the past decade, new versions have emerged that consider biopsychosocial factors such as belief as having a more proactive role in the presentation of illness, recovery and probability of return to work (Waddell, 1998; Munitz and Rudnick, 2000). Central to these revisions is the assumption that disease and illness do not exclusively result from demonstrable patho-physiology but may crucially involve and can be meaningfully explained in terms of psychological and socio-cultural factors (Wade and Halligan, 2004).

The conference on which this book was based provided an opportunity to probe deeper into the nature of beliefs and in particular to collate and highlight theoretical vocational and clinical reports demonstrating the significant role that beliefs play in defining and understanding illness presentation, compliance with treatment, disability and return to work (Horne, 1999; Gupta and Home 2001; Haynes *et al.*, 1978; Waddell and Alyward, 2005).

Nature of beliefs

Paraphrasing William James, we all know what beliefs are – so long as no one asks us to define them. Beliefs however are as real as other social constructs and exist because most people tacitly agree to act as if they exist. Unlike other social constructions such as money, freewill and citizenship, beliefs refer to a category of personal truth or implicit theory whose main function is to provide meaning and certainty 'about matters that have to do with the ideas we hold of ourselves' (Damasio, 2000). However, like other cognitive processes, we possess little introspective knowledge of the preconscious processing involved in belief formation (Halligan and Oakley, 2000). Moreover, intuitive experience suggests that we do not consciously choose our beliefs and 'it is likely that the mechanisms which allow us to develop the basis of beliefs, as well as the mechanisms by which we retrieve and express them, are operated in a largely covert manner' (Damasio, 2000).

Unlike other mental constructs, beliefs are powerful precisely because they provide the 'mental scaffolding' for appraising, explaining and integrating new observations; in other words, making sense of where we are, what we are about, and collectively providing a steadfast guide to managing the world in which we find ourselves. According to Dennett (1987), beliefs can be considered the inner causes that provide for describing and predicting a person's behaviour (what he calls 'taking the intentional stance'). To say that someone believes something is [to say that] that someone is disposed to behave in a certain way under certain conditions.

From a psychological perspective, beliefs remain crucial components of personality and the sense of identity used to define the way others see us. Significantly, many of our attitudes (mental dispositions to act), established ways of responding to people and situations, utterances and ability to cope (Lazarus and Folkman 1984) can be attributed to implicit or explicitly held beliefs. Indeed, it is not possible to understand racism, bias, superstition, prejudice, religious persecution and political conflict without considering disagreement within basic ontological belief systems.

One has only to think of the extraordinary influence that Copernicus' theories, Newton's physics and Darwin's Evolutionism have had in challenging and revising existing beliefs in the history of human knowledge to recognise how shared pre-existing notions of the world and human nature can determine and constrain interpretations and explanations. In medicine, reductionism (symptoms as inevitable indices of disease) and dualism (physical (ie bodily) related ailments most preferentially distinguised from mental symptoms) continue to characterize assesments and interventions (Borrell-Carrio, Suchnan, Epstein (2004). What about Psychology? For much of the early half of the 20th century, many psychologists accepted (believed?) what would be considered today a radical behaviourist position – namely that observable behaviour is *all* there is to mental life. This approach considered behaviour as the product of conditioned mental processes and, as such, thoughts, feelings and intentions were largely superfluous for the purposes of psychological research. The subsequent computational view of the human mind as an information processor (cognitive science) in the 1960's facilitated a move towards a re-examination of those inner structures and processors while employing the scientific trappings of experimentation. However, religous beliefs are perhaps the best examples of how powerful predispositions can govern and influence behaviour.

Many millions worldwide who claim commitment to formal religions (presumably) hold beliefs regarding the particular nature of the supernatural, morality, values, and associated rituals to justify and differentiate their respective adherence. In America, large scale representative polls consistently show that 90% of the population claim a belief in God, with a sizeable majority also reporting a believe that God takes a personal interest in their lives and intervenes to help them. Consequently 'when President Bush said, "God told me to strike at al-Qaeda and I struck them, and then he instructed me to strike at Saddam, which I did," most Americans were not alarmed to learn that their leader was receiving orders that no one else could hear' (Gilbert, 2005). According to Humphrey (1997), '[the] problem is not just that so many adults believe in things that flatly contradict the modern scientific world but that so many do not believe in things that are absolutely central to the scientific view'. Examples of the latter include survey findings which found that less than 50% believed in human evolution and that less than 10% believe that evolution – even if it did occur – could have taken place without some form of external intervention. In California religious fundamentalists successfully lobbied for restrictions on the teaching of Darwinian evolution in public school textbooks (Gilbert, 1993).

Beliefs also provide for expectancies and hence their influence is not only retrospective but, more critically one that shapes on-line experiences including the experience and interpretation of symptoms (Kuhner& Raetzke, 1989; Horn, James, Petrie, Weinman & Vincent, 2000). How can pre-existing notions influence our perceptions/experience?

Visual illusions provide a useful illustration. Here the interpretation (final perception) of an object or scene is not determined solely by the empirical sensory information formed on the retina. Illusions, by definition, refer to perceptions that do not correspond to what is actually in the real world but perceptions that we are convinced are true nevertheless. Illusions are basically the result of 'top-down' built-in bias or predispositions as to how to see the world. The Müller-Lyer illusion (Figure 1) is a good illustration of how such a predisposition towards perceiving an apparent line-length difference remains stable and enduring over time. Even when you *know* that both of the horizontal lines are the same length, an uncontrollable consequence of the visual representation requires one to consciously reject this proposition (Bever, 1986).

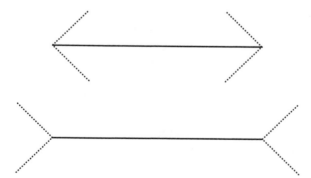

Figure 1 Müller-Lyer illusion

A similar reconstructive account has been put forward to explain the expected or predicted sensory feedback generated when we initiate planned limb movements (Wolpert, 1997). When moving a limb, sensory information (derived from current state information including the alignment of joints prior to initiation of a motor command) appears crucial for deciding the type and extent of proprioceptive awareness that is associated with the intended movement. This information is thought to arise from a 'feed forward' system which predicts the sensory consequences of a motor command and is monitored directly by comparing the predicted movements with those of actual sensory feedback (Wolpert et al., 1995). According to this account, every time a motor command is issued to a limb, an 'efference copy' of that motor command (a predicted or expected somatosensory experience) is produced in parallel. According to Frith *et al.* (2000), our normal awareness and experience of our limb movement (given the latency in translating online information) is largely based on this predicted state rather than the actual feedback state, unless the system monitoring the actual feedback detects a deviation from that predicted. In patients after limb amputation, such motor commands when issued in most cases produce a discernable experience of limbless perception often described as a phantom limb moving (Halligan, 2002). Conversely, when the motor command is not accompanied by confirmatory feedback from the efference copy, as appears to be the case in some hypnotically suggested 'automatic' limb movements, the self-generated action is experienced (falsely) as a passive movement caused by an external agency (Blakemore, Oakley and Frith, 2003).

The idea that much of our phenomenological experience is the product of hidden *reconstructive* top-down processes rather than the translation of sensory transducers was one of the key features of cognitive psychology following the collapse of behaviourism in the 1950s. In the case of vision, this constructive account suggests that everything seen is a construct (product) of the brain's interpretation of the sensory input. This includes colour, shading, texture, motion, shape, visual objects – the entire visual scene. (Hoffman, 1998). Experience is therefore not simply the registration of 'pure sensory experience' but rather the constructive integration of sensory information filtered through 'predictive brain-based hypotheses' regarding what is out there. This interpretative filter provides for the meaning, structure and unity of immediate experience (Gregory, 1998) and has still to be fully appreciated within cognitive neuroscience (Hassin, Uleman and Bargh, 2005).

As such, believing can be considered analogous to seeing, however since not all seeing produces an accurate picture of reality, knowing the role beliefs play is important as we tend not to look for things that we don't expect (i.e. believe in). Having a belief changes the way evidence is collected and evaluated (Reisberg, Pearson and Kosslyn, 2003; Vincete and Brewer 1993). The tendency to evaluate incoming evidence in support of current beliefs when new evidence is encountered has serious consequences. Carlson and Russo (2001) showed that 'predecisional distortion' in potential jurors meant that they were highly susceptible to arriving at unfair verdicts due, in the main, to the tendency to view each new piece of evidence with a bias toward the party that the juror already favoured. Carlson and Russo (2001) maintain 'that people create narratives based on their own experiences to make the facts of a case understandable to themselves'.

Two clinical examples illustrate the way in which top-down or pre-existing notions may shape experience and expectation. The first concerns the way in which prior information can bias symptom symptom interpretation. In one study, twenty neurologists were asked to judge a number of plantar responses from film (two of which showed equivocal toe movements presented twice at the same sitting with a fictitious history and examination results (minus the plantar reflex). Van Gijn & Bonke (1977) showed that the neurologist's interpretation of the two equivocal toe movements were biased significantly (P < 0.01) according to the clinical information provided. Thirty different neurologists who rated the two films without clinical data did not show this bias.

The second example involved a study by Mittenberg, diGiulio, Perrin and Bass designed to see whether symptoms of mild brain damage could be related to what patients believed to be the likely symptoms to follow head injury. In this novel study, Mittenberg *et al.* (1992) asked 223 controls with no personal experience or knowledge of head injury to complete an affective, somatic, and memory check-list as to their expectations of symptoms 6 months post head injury. A similar checklist was given to 100 patients with head injuries for comparison. Predicted concussion symptoms in the naïve controls reliably showed a coherent cluster of symptoms virtually identical to the post-concussion syndrome reported by patients with head trauma, suggesting a possible aetiological role for expectations in the experience and expression of symptoms. Patients, on the other hand, consistently underestimated the pre-morbid prevalence of the symptoms compared with controls.

Exploring beliefs

According to **Bell, Halligan and Ellis, (Chapter 1)** the absence of a formally agreed or accepted definition of belief has hindered the formal cognitive /psychological study of beliefs by comparison with other well developed areas of cognitive neuroscience such as attention, memory and language. In psychiatry, delusions are traditionally considered 'pathological beliefs', although existing cognitive approaches differ in their willingness to explain delusions solely in terms of an impairment model of normal belief formation (Bell, Halligan and Ellis 2003). Nevertheless, the chapter by Bell et al. which focuses on the study of paranormal beliefs and mono-thematic delusions, provides a comprehensive review of the current psychological and psychiatric accounts, while highlighting some of the recent candidate cognitive processes thought to be involved. Although it is unlikely that a unitary belief formation process will be formulated on the basis of the neuropsychological evidence alone, this productive vein of research has already yielded several interesting leads.

The question remains however, why some people come to believe certain ideas (i.e. hold them as true) and not others. There is growing evidence that people have a tendency to believe what they should not (Gilbert, 1991).

Apparently, 'repeated exposure to assertions for which there is no evidence increases the likelihood that people will believe those assertions' (Gilbert et al., 1993). In addition, 'several studies have suggested that under some circumstances, people will believe assertions that are explicitly labelled as false'(Gilbert *et al.*, 1993).

In **Chapter 2, Marks** describes research on the fascinating phenomenon of 'subjective validation' or the 'personal validation effect'. This reliable but striking effect provides some insight into the high levels of belief in the paranormal within society. Beliefs in the paranormal have always been a relevant and fertile source of investigation for researchers interested in understanding belief formation and its resilience to enquiry (Lawrence & Peters, 2004). In particular, there is no shortage of opinion polls that reliably report that a majority of people believe in angels, life after death and extraterrestrials. According to a recent Mori poll survey (August, 2003) a representative crosssection of the British public (N = 1001) show high levels of belief in the paranormal: 64% believe in God; 47% believe in life after death; 68% believe in a soul; 38% believe in ghosts; 51% believe in telepathy and 51% believe in extra-sensory perception.

Initially described by the psychologist, Bertram Forer the 'personal validation effect' arose from the observation that people tend to accept vague and general personality descriptions as uniquely applicable to themselves without realizing that the same description could just as easily be applied to anyone. As a form of 'confirmation bias', the personal validation effect essentially works because supporting data is more heavily weighted than disconfirming data. As a result, most people can be persuaded into believing that they are right even when the evidence points towards the possibility that they are wrong. In his own research designed to reveal the psychological characteristics of people who believe or not in psychic phenomena, Marks found that believers showed a strong tendency to subjectively validate and tended to exhibit personality characteristics linked to schizotypy.

In **Chapter 3, Deeley** considers beliefs about illness and its treatment from a 'cognitive anthropological perspective' and shows that there is considerable scope for productive dialogue between anthropology and cognitive science, particularly in relation to how group level processes may contribute to cognition. The challenge remains to integrate the experimental approach of cognitive science with the anthropological tradition of describing and interpreting the complex social and informational environments that human beings inhabit. The value of anthropological accounts is that they draw attention to how fractionated cognitive processes, including those underlying beliefs, are functionally integrated to support locally coherent and meaningful participation in diverse social contexts (Deeley, 1999).

The extent to which beliefs can colour expectations and confound treatment outcome (e.g. selection bias, observer bias, reporting bias and reviewer bias) has been well established in medicine (Sackett, 1979; Jadad *et al.* 1996). Schultz, *et al.*, (1995) found that non-randomised studies compared to studies that employed adequately concealed treatment allocations, tended to overestimate treatment effect, by 41%. The same study reported that non-blinded studies over-estimated treatment effects by about 17%. Cultural aspects are also implicated. Vickers *et al.*, (1995) showed that acupuncture trials conducted in east Asia were always positive, whereas similar trials in Australia/New Zealand, north America or western Europe were only positive half the time.

Awareness that the beliefs/interests of those taking part and organizing clinical trials can confound or prejudice the interpretation and significance of results has been a key motivating factor behind improvements to research design in modem medicine (including the use of double blind randomised control trials, systematic reviews and more recently the formal journal policy requiring conflict of interest declarations).

More difficult to control however has been publication bias (Cowley, Skene, Stainer & Hampton, 1993). To rectify this, several leading medical journals recently agreed that they will now only consider trials for publication that have been registered in a trial registry (Eysenbach, 2004). The growing close financial relationship between academia and industry provide, yet a further base for potential bias (Angell, 2000). Despite attempting to minimize the potential adverse influence that subjective predispositions (beliefs) may have on medical judgements and decisions in formal clinical trials, there are few explicit attempts to control for this naturalistic and prevalent human character in everyday medical practice.

In drug trials, the placebo response is the best known and perhaps best-studied example of the power of patient belief (Harrington, 1999). Indeed, placebo effects are sufficiently powerful that they have been shown to reverse the effect of active drugs (Wolf, 1950). In **Chapter 4, Irving Kirsch** reviews the evidence illustrating the power of placebos and their phenomenal ability to affect physical and emotional responses. Starting with Parkinson's disease, where long-standing effects have been shown on objective motor performance and even neuroimaging studies, the placebo response is equal to that of the active drug apomorphine. Similar accounts are described for rheumatoid arthritis, asthma, contact dermatitis and sexual dysfunction. However, it is in the areas of pain, anxiety and depression that the effects of placebos have been well established (Kirsch *et al.*, 2002). An outstanding problem, however, remains how to prescribe placebos without deception, particularly in situations where an active treatment is neither available nor advisable.

Significance of beliefs

What people believe about the nature of their illness and its presentation affects how both they and their doctors cope and deal with it (Furze *et al.*, 2002; Bates *et al.*, 1997; Stroud *et al.*, 2000). Knowing a patient's beliefs regarding their condition (their illness representation) is clinically relevant for managing their condition. Knowing a patient's belief can predict their subjective experience, capacity to cope, recovery (Diefenbach & Leventhal, 1996), treatment compliance and behaviour (Weinman and Petrie, 1997). After stroke, negative attitudes and beliefs have been associated with length of survival (Lewis Dennis, O'Rourke & Sharpe, 2001) and has been shown to thought to hinder recovery, while positive beliefs are associated more with improvements in functional outcome (Watson Haviland, Greer, Davidson & Bliss, 2002). Patients' beliefs concerning the causes and prognoses of their illnesses (with and without evidence of organic pathophysiology) remain fundamental for a number of theoretical models of illness behaviour (Rosenstock, 1974; Wade and Halligan, 2003) causation (Srinivasan & Thara, 2001) and medication compliance (Horne *et al.*, 1999).

In the case of pain, patients' initial beliefs about the success of a given treatment have been shown to have an important influence on final treatment outcome and adjustment to chronic pain (Stroud *et al.*, 2000). Goossens *et al.* (2005) recently showed that pre-treatment expectancy significantly predicted outcome immediately after treatment and at 12 months follow-up in the case of a cognitive-behavioural intervention for patients with chronic musculoskeletal pain. Patients who seem to be more positive about their future have a much better functional outcome than those who hold negative beliefs about their illness and recovery. Using the Illness Representation Questionnaire (IPQ) Vaughan, Morrison & Miller (2003) found that illness beliefs had a direct effect on functional outcome in patients with MS. These studies further highlight the importance of providing suitable interventions to modify illness cognitions which have shown to be related to poor outcomes. In the case of Rheumatoid Arthritis (RA), illness perceptions have significant implications for adaptation to illness and they often outweigh the impact of medical disease status on depression, physical function and pain (Groarke *et al.*, 2004).

In **Chapter 5, Ferrari, Kwan & Friel** explore the changing concept and beliefs relating to the sick role. Traditionally considered a role for which the patient is not responsible (Parson, 1951), they argue that while society accepts that the pain in rheumatoid arthritis is something beyond one's control, if a 'disease' is not proven then society does not always share this view. The rise in symptom based conditions has provided for the growth of many 'controversial disability syndromes' and with it, the exploration of non-medical alternatives (Halligan *et al.*, 2003) for illness behaviours that consider volitional control a legitimate causal contributing factor. While agreeing that belief systems clearly influence the behaviour of many chronic pain patients, Ferrari et al. suggest that such belief systems operate at both a preconscious and conscious volitional level. In their chapter, they review historical examples where clinicians have begun to explore the role of volition in illness behaviour to better understand chronic whiplash syndrome.

Drawing on his own clinical experience, **Wade** in **Chapter 6** considers the role of beliefs and associated expectations in explaining successful patient participation in and outcome of rehabilitation. Research studies confirm the importance of belief for both prognosis and effectiveness of rehabilitation (Petrie *et al.*, 1996). Indeed, Wade suggests that the effectiveness of rehabilitation could be increased through harnessing the power of belief. A striking example is the study by Moffet *et al.* (2005) where the patient's belief in the efficacy of therapy for back pain was noted to strongly influence the extent of response. In the case of chronic fatigue, Sharpe *et al.* (1996) have shown that cognitive behavioural treatment directed at helping patients to re-evaluate their understanding of the illness and to adopt more effective coping behaviours resulted in a sustained reduction in functional impairment. Wade goes further and suggests that beliefs held by significant others also need to be considered and in particular the beliefs and expectations of family members and purchasers of rehabilitation services. Within the rehabilitation process, he suggests that we should consider explicitly manipulating the patient's expectations to improve their outcome while at the same time attempting to alter societal beliefs about rehabilitation.

Despite growing evidence for specific new interventions, Wade and DeJong (2000) have suggested that the major advances over the past decade have been more conceptual rather than practical. In particular, they suggest that the revised ICIDH model has facilitated a change of emphasis within rehabilitation from a predominantly medical one to one in which psychological and socio-cultural aspects are equally important. Current evidence indicates that the provision of a multidisciplinary rehabilitation service actually improves recovery (Ottenbacher and Jannell, 1993; SUTC, 1997). However, explanations for this consistent finding remain unclear since the stroke units in question did not routinely employ any medical or surgical interventions that might be expected to influence the pathological process or immediate neurological complications of stroke disease (SUTC, 1997). One possibility for the relative success of stroke units operating 'a more coordinated and focused program of rehabilitation' is the extent to which the multidisciplinary rehabilitation process facilitated shared beliefs within staff and patients as regards knowledge of the illness, prognosis and interventions involved. Such an approach provides for the rehabilitation process to continue therapeutic strategies beyond formal therapy sessions thereby allowing patients to achieve greater independence.

Locating illness and disability within a social context

As a subjective state of feeling unwell, illness is culturally defined and socially sanctioned – as such – traditional reductionist biomedical models will always struggle to provide satisfactory explanations for the patient or clinician (Barsky and Borus, 1999; Sharpe and Carson, 2001; Wade and Halligan, 2004). Over the past two decades, a widening gulf has emerged between illness presentation and the adequacy of traditional biomedical explanations – all of which reinforce the fact that illness is socially and culturally embedded. Moreover, traditional healthcare 'can do little in the face of the social reality of a chosen lifestyle or destructive behaviour' (Malleson, 2002). The focus on psychosocial factors is timely, given the growing levels of disability, creeping medicalisation (Moynihan, Health and Henry, 2002, Hadler, 2004), and 'diagnostic creep' (Farah, 2002) together with the increasing numbers of patients who now present with disabling and often unexplained somatic and mental symptoms where no relevant pathology or known psychopathology can be established (Kirmayer et al., 2004).

To bridge this gap, health care professionals from different sectors of medicine have begun to consider the biopsychosocial (BPS) approach (Engel 1977; Waddell et al., 2004; Kiesler 1999; White 2005). Psychosocial factors such as beliefs are particularly relevant when one considers the prevalent notions (potential biases) harboured within medicine and society regarding the causes of illness, expected recovery and medication efficiency (see chapters by Horne (Chapter 8), Jorm (Chapter 7), Burton et al. (Chapter 10) & Buchbinder (Chapter 11). For example, it is widely assumed (believed) that medical practice during the 19/20th centuries played a decisive role in halting or reducing the major mortality based diseases such as whooping cough, scarlet fever, measles, tuberculosis and typhoid fever. However as Malleson (2002) points out, most of these conditions 'had already stopped being major killers before effective medical interventions were introduced for either their cure or their intervention..[and hence] it was social factors and not medical care that transformed . . . [these] health statistics'.

In addition it is important to recognize that illness beliefs are and never were the preserve of the patient, but crucially depends on the views of all health care professionals and society involved which dynamically contribute to the interpretations of symptoms, patient presentation and treatment outcomes (Cherkin et al., 1995). The physician's own 'behaviour can be influenced by patient expectations and other psychosocial factors (Buchbinder et al., 2001). In reviewing the Australian epidemic of repetitive strain injury (RSI) in the early 1980's (where

New South Wales saw an eleven-fold increase in disability claims), Lucire (2003) argued that doctors played an important (if unknowing) part in the belief that RSI was the primary result of an occupational injury caused by inhumane working conditions (Elliot, 2004). Hadler (2004) goes even further and suggests that the "wealth of health information promulgated by all sorts of PURUEYORS of health care including the medical profession [although] . . . intended to be helpful . . . destroys our sense of invincibility, without doing much for either our health or our lorgevity.

An adequate understanding of illness and disability can no longer ignore the (often implicit) beliefs held by healthcare professionals, academics and those in wider society regarding the causes of illness, the extent of disability, recovery and the potential for treatment. Future developments of the biopsychosocial model need to take account of the beliefs of all the key players involved. Central to this account is the 'view that [all] individuals construct models, internal representations or schema which reflect their pooled understanding of previous experiences and [these] are used for interpreting new ones and planning behaviour' (Weinman and Petrie, 1997). As a social organisations, healthcare systems depend on members of society adopting a congruent belief system (model) regarding the expectations and responsibilities associated with illness and the sick role (see Aylward, 2006). Wade and Halligan (2004) suggest that the adoption and use of a psychosocial model would improve the delivery of better health care more than any other change in healthcare organisation. This remains the challenge.

The growing research on beliefs highlighted in this book will hopefully invigorate and extend emerging biopsychosocial models of illness (see White, 2005).

References

Angell M (2000). Is Academic Medicine for Sale? *New England Journal of Medicine* **342**: 1516–1518.

Aylward M (2006). Belief: Clinical and Vocational Interventions. In P.W. Halligan and M. Aylward (eds) *The Power of Belief*. Oxford University Press.

Aylward M and LoCascio J (1995). 'Problems in the Assessment of Psychosomatic Conditions in Social Security Benefits and Related Commercial Schemes'. In: *Journal of Psychosomatic Research*, **39**(6): 755–765.

Barsky AD and Borus JF (1999). Functional Somatic Syndromes. Volume 130, Issue 11, pp910–921.

Bates MS, Rankin-Hill L, and Sanchez-Ayendez M (1997). The effects of cultural context of health care on treatment and response to chronic pain and illness. *Soc Sci Med.*, **45**: 1433–1447.

Bell V, Halligan PW, and Ellis HD (2006). A Cognitive Neuroscience of Belief. In P.W. Halligan and M. Aylward (eds) *The Power of Belief*. Oxford: Oxford University Press.

Bell V, Halligan PW, and Ellis HD (2003). Beliefs About Delusions. *The Psychologist*, **16** (8): 418–423.

Bever TG (1986). The Aesthetic Basis for Cognitive Structures. In M. Brand and R.M. Harnish *The representation of knowledge and belief*, pp314–356, Tuscon: University of Arizona Press.

Blakemore S-J, Oakley DA, and Frith CD (2003). Delusions of alien control in the normal brain, *Neuropsychologia*, **41**: 1058–1067.

Borrell-Carrio F, Suchman AL, and Epstein RM (2004). The Biopsychological Model 25 years later: Principles, Practice, and Scientific inquiry. *Annals of Family Medicine* **2**: 576–582.

Buchbinder R, Jolley D, and Wyatt M (2001). Population based intervention to change back pain beliefs and disability: three part evaluation. *BMJ.* **322**(7301): 1516–1520.

Carlson J and Russo E (2001). Biased Interpretation of Evidence by Mock Jurors. *Journal of Experimental Psychology*: Applied 2001, Vol 7, No. 2,91–103.

Cherkin DC, Deyo RA, Wheeler K, and Ciol MA (1995). Physician views about treating low back pain. The results of a national survey. *Spine*, 1;**20**(1): l–9.

Cowley AJ, Skene A, Stainer K, and Hampton JR (1993). The effect of lorcainide on arrhythmias and survival in patients with acute myocardial infarction: an example of publication bias. *Int J Cardiol*, **40**(2): 161–166.

Damasio AR (2000). Thinking about Belief: concluding remarks. In Daniel L. Schacter and Elaine Scarry (ed.)*Memory, Brain and Belief*. Cambridge, MA: Harvard University Press.

Deeley PQ (1999). Ecological Understandings of Mental and Physical Illness. *Philosophy, Psychiatry and Psychology*, **6**(2).

Dennett D (1987). *The Intentional Stance*. The MIT Press.

Diefenbach MA and Leventhal H (1996). The common sense model of illness representation: theoretical and practical consideration. *J Soc Distress Homeless*, **5**: 11–38.

Elliot C (2004). Scrivener's Palsy, London Review of Books, Vol. 26 No. 1.

Engel GL (1977). The need for a new medical model: A challenge for biomedicine. *Science*, **196**(4286): 129–136.

Eysenbach G (2004). Tackling Publication Bias and Selective Reporting in Health Informatics Research: Register your eHealth Trials in the International eHealth Studies Registry *J Med Internet Research*, **6**(3): e35.

Farah MJ (2002). Emerging ethical issues in neuroscience. *Nature Neuroscience.* **5**(11): 1123–1129.

Forer BR (1949). 'The Fallacy of Personal Validation: A classroom demonstration of gullibility'. *Journal of Abnormal Psychology*, **44**: 118–121.

Frith CD, Blakemore SJ, and Wolpert DM (2000). Abnormalities in the awareness and control of action. *Philosl Trans R Soc Lond B Biol Sci*, **355**: 1771–1788.

Furze G, Roebuck A, Bull P, Lewin RJP, and Thompson DR (2002). A comparison of the illness beliefs of people with angina and their peers: a questionnaire study. *BMC Cardiovascular Disorders*, **2**(4).

Gilbert DT, Tafarodi RW, and Malone PS (1993). You can't not believe everything you read. *J Pers Soc Psychol*, **65**(2): 221–233.

Gilbert DT (1991). How mental systems believe. *American Psychologist*, **46**: 107–119.

Gilbert P (1995). Biopsychosocial approaches and evolutionary theory as aids to integration in clinical psychology and psychotherapy. *Clinical Psychology and Psychotherapy*, **2**: 135–156.

Gilbert P (2002). Understanding the biopsychosocial approach: Conceptualization. *Clinical Psychology,* **14**: 13–17

Gilbert DT (2005). The vagaries of religious experience, *Edge,* September.

Goossens ME, Vlaeyen JW, Hidding A, Kole-Snijders A, and Evers SM (2005). Treatment expectancy affects the outcome of cognitive-behavioural interventions in chronic pain. *Clin J Pain,* **21**(1): 18–26.

Green CD (1995, August). Foucault and folk psychology. In C. D. Green (Chair), *Postmodernism and cognitive science.* Organizer and chair of symposium conducted at the annual conference of the American Psychological Association, New York, New York.

Gregory R (1998). Brainy mind. *British Medical Journal,* **317**(7174): 1693–1695.

Groarke A, Curtis R, Coughlan R, and Gsel A (2004). The role of perceived and actual disease status in adjustment to rheumatoid arthritis. *Rheumatology,* **43**: 1142–1149.

Gupta K and Home R (2001). The influence of health beliefs on the presentation and consultation outcome in patients with chemical sensitivities. *Journal of Psychosomatic Research,* **50**: 131–137.

Hadler NM (2004). *The Last Well Person.* McGill-Queen's University Press, Montreal.

Halligan PW (eds) (2002). Phantom limbs: The body in mind. *Cogntive Neuropsychiatry,* **7**(3): 251–268.

Halligan PW, Bass C, and Oakley DA (eds.) (2003). *Malingering and Illness Deception.* Oxford University Press, UK.

Halligan PW and Oakley D (2000). Greatest Myth of All. *New Scientist,* 2265, 34–39.

Harrington A (eds.) (1999). *The Placebo Effect: An interdisciplinary exploration.* Harvard University Press.

Hassin RR, Uleman JS, and Bargh JA (eds.) (2005). *The new unconscious.* New York: Oxford University Press.

Haynes RB, Taylor DW, and Sackett DL (1979). *Compliance in Healthcare.* Baltimore, Maryland: USA: John Hopkins University Press.

Haynes RB, Sackett DL, Taylor DW, Gibson ES, and Johnson AL (1978). Increased absenteeism from work after detection and labeling of hypertensive patients. *N Engl J Med.* **299**(14): 741–744.

Hoffman DD (1998). *Visual Intelligence.* New York and London, Norton and Company

Horne R, Graupner L, Frost S, Weinman J, Wright SM, and Hankins M (2004). Medicine in a multi-cultural society: the effect of cultural background on beliefs about medications. *Soc SciMed.* **59**(6): 1307–1313.

Horne R, James D, Petrie K, Weinman J, and Vincent R (2000). Patients' interpretation of symptoms as a cause of delay in reaching hospital during acute myocardial infarction. *Heart.* **83**(4): 388–393.

Horne R (1999). Patients' beliefs about treatment: the hidden determinant of treatment outcome? *Journal of Psychosomatic Research,* **47**: 491–495.

Humphrey N (1998). What shall we tell the children? Oxford Amnesty Lecture. *Social Research,* **65**: 777–805.

Janz NK and Becker MH (1984). The health belief model: A decade later. *Health Education Quarterly,* **11**(1): 1–47.

Jadad AR, and McQuay HJ (1996). Meta-analysis to evaluate analgesic interventions: a systematic qualitative review of the literature. *J Clin Epidemiol,* **49**: 235–243.

Kiesler DJ (1999). *Beyond the Disease Model of Mental Disorders.* New York, Praeger.

Kirmayer LJ, Groleau D, Looper KJ, and Dao MD (2004). Explaining medically unexplained symptoms. *Can J Psychiatry*. **49**(10): 663–672.

Kirsch I (2006). Placebo: the role of expectancies in the generation and alleviation of illness. In P.W. Halligan and M. Aylward (eds) *The Power of Belief*. Oxford: Oxford University Press.

Kirsch I, Moore TJ, Scoboria A, and Nicholls SS (2002). The emperor's new drugs: an analysis of antidepressant medication data submitted to the US Food and Drug Administration. *Prevention and Treatment*, **5**(23).

Kuhner MK and Raetzke PB (1989). The effect of health beliefs on the compliance of periodontal patients with oral hygiene instructions. *J Periodontol*. **60**(1): 51–56.

Lazarus RS and Folkman S (1984). *Stress, Appraisal, and Coping*. New York: Springer.

Lawrence E and Peters E (2004). Reasoning in believers in the paranormal. *Journal of Nerv Ment Dis*, **192**(11): 727–733.

Lewis SC, Dennis MS, O'Rourke SJ, and Sharpe M (2001). Negative attitudes among short-term stroke survivors predict worse long-term survival. *Stroke* **32**: 1640–1645.

Lucire Y (2003). *Constructing RSI: Belief and Desire*. UNSW PRESS.

Marks D (in press). Biased beliefs and the subjective validation effect. In PW Halligan and Aylward M (eds.) The Power of Belief. Oxford: Oxford University Press.

Malleson A (2002). Whiplash and other useful illnesses. McGill-Queens University Press, Montreal.

Mittenberg W, DiGiulio DV, Perrin S, and Bass AE (1992). Symptoms following mild head injury: expectation as aetiology. *Journal of neurology, neurosurgery and psychiatry*, **55**: 200–204.

Moffett JAK, Jackson DA, Richmond S, Hanh S, Coulton S, Farrin A, Manca A, and Torgerson DJ (2005). Randomised trial of a brief physiotherapy intervention compared with usual physiotherapy for neck pain patients: outcomes and patients' preference. *British Medical Journal*, 8; **330**(7482): 75.

Moynihan R, Heath I, and Henry D (2002). Selling sickness: the pharmaceutical industry and disease mongering. *BMJ*, **324**: 886–891.

Munitz H, Rudnick A (2000). The biopsychosocial model of medicine revisited: a meta-theoretical excursion. *Israel Journal of Psychiatry*, **37**: 266–270.

Ogden J (2004). *Health Psychology*, 3rd edition, Open University Press: Buckingham.

Ottenbacher KJ and Jannell S (1993). The results of clinical trials in stroke rehabilitation research. *Arch Neurology*, **50**(1): 37–44.

Petrie KJ, Weinman J, Sharpe N, and Buckley J (1996). Role of patients' view of their illness in predicting return to work and functioning after myocardial infarction: longitudinal study. *British Medical Journal* 11; **312**: 1191–1194.

Parsons and Talcott (1951). *The Social System*. Free Press.

Reisberg D, Pearson DG, and Kosslyn SM (2003). Institutions and introspection's about imagery: the role of imagery experience in shaping an investigator's theoretical views. *Applied Cognitive Psychology*, **17**: 147–160

Rosenstock (1974). Historical Origins of the Health Belief Model. *Health Education Monographs*. Vol. 2 No. 4.

Sackett DL (1979). Bias in analytic research. *Journal of Chronic Diseases*, **32**: 51–63.

Sharpe M, Hawton K, Simkin S, Surawy C, Hackmann A, Klimes I, Peto T, Warrell D, and Seagroatt V (1996). Cognitive behaviour therapy for the chronic fatigue syndrome: a randomized controlled trial. *BMJ*, 6; **312**: 22–26.

Sharpe M and Carson A (2001). 'Unexplained somatic symptoms, functional syndromes, and somatization: do we need a paradigm shift?' *Annals of internal medicine*, **134**: 926–930.

Schultz KF, Chalmers I, Hayes RJ, and Altman DG (1995). Empirical evidence of bias: Dimensions of methodological quality associated with estimates of treatment effects in controlled trials. *Journal of the American Medical Association*, **273**: 408–412.

Srinivasan TN and Thara R (2001). Beliefs about causation of schizophrenia: do Indian families believe in supernatural causes? *Soc Psychiatry Psychiatr Epidemiol*, **36**(3): 134–140.

Stroke Unit Trialists' Collaboration [**SUTC**] (1997). Collaborative systematic review of the randomised trials of organised inpatient (stroke unit) care after stroke. *BMJ*, **314**: 1151 (19 April).

Stroud MW, Thorn BE, Jensen MP, and Boothby JL (2000). The relation between pain beliefs, negative thoughts, and psychosocial functioning in chronic pain patients. *Pain*, **84**(2–3): 347–352.

Van Gijn J and Bonke B (1977). Interpretation of plantar reflexes: biasing effect of other signs and symptoms. *Journal of Neurology, Neurosurgery and Psychiatry*, **40**: 787–789.

Vaughan R, Morrison L, and Miller E (2003). The illness representations of multiple sclerosis and their relations to outcome. *British Journal of Health Psychology*, **8**: 287–301.

Vicente KJ and Brewer WF (1993). Reconstructive remembering of the scientific literature. *Cognition*, **46**(2): 101–128.

Waddell G and Aylward M (2005). *The scientific and conceptual basis of incapacity benefits*. The Stationery Office, London.

Waddell G *The back pain revolution*. Churchill Livingstone, Edinburgh. Second Edition 2004.

Wade DT (2006). Beliefs in rehabilitation, the hidden power for change. In PW Halligan and M Aylward (eds.) *The Power of Belief*. Oxford: Oxford University Press.

Wade DT and Halligan PW (2004). Do biomedical models of illness make for good healthcare systems? *BMJ*, 11;**329**(7479): 1398–1401.

Wade DT and de Jong BA (2000). Recent advances in rehabilitation. *BMJ*, **320**(7246): 1385–1388.

Wade DT and Halligan PW (2003). New wine in old bottles: the WHO ICF as an explanatory model of human behaviour. *Clinical Rehabilitation*, **17**(4): 349–354.

Watson M, Haviland J, Greer S, Davidson J, and Bliss J (1999). Influence of psychological response on survival in breast cancer: a population-based cohort study. *The Lancet*, **9187**: 1331–1336.

Weinman J and Petrie KJ (1997). Illness perceptions: a new paradigm for psychosomatics? *J Psychosom Res.*, **42**(2): 113–116.

White P (2005). *Biopsychosocial Medicine*: An integrated approach to understanding illness. Oxford University Press.

Vickers A, Goyal N, Harland R, and Rees R (1998). Do certain countries produce only positive results? A systematic review of controlled trials. *Controlled Clinical Trials*, **19**: 159–166.

Wolf S (1950). Effects of suggestion and conditioning on the action of chemical agents in human subjects: the pharmacology of placebos. *Journal of Clinical Investigation*, **29**: 100–109

Wolpert DM (1997). Computational approaches to motor control. *Trends Cognit Sci*, **1**(6): 209–216.

Wolpert DM, Ghahramani Z, and Jordan MI (1995). An internal model for sensorimotor integration. *Science*, **269**: 1880–1882.

Beliefs: Clinical and vocational interventions; tackling psychological and social determinants of illness and disability

Mansel Aylward

A simple definition of belief might be that it is something that one holds to be true. Though naive this critical aspect has a common-sense ring to it. Why not adopt this simple approach from the outset? Surely a description or definition of a belief needs to be based on such common-sense understanding and usage of everyday language. But common-sense and scientific description are rarely good bedfellows. However even if we adopt this simple common sense approach to the meaning of 'belief:', which reflects its everyday use, it is difficult to argue that beliefs do not constitute one of the most important determinants, if not the principal source, of human behaviour. Our beliefs continue to be powerful and relevant drives of human behaviour and constitute a central component of the biopsychosocial approach to explaining illness behaviours. (White 2005).

What then is a belief? If the study of cognition is to understand the way human beings perceive and learn, reason and think, and imagine (George 1962), then the formulation of beliefs as a unique form of the cognitive process also need to be considered. So belief must be some sort of association held in the mind and gained through experience of some internal or external stimuli which predicts a particular outcome or response. Presumably, then, the acquisition of beliefs comes about by the accumulation of these associations with the usual outcome or outcomes over time. On that premise, acquisition of beliefs would involve many associations based on many experiences. In this context, the stored associations should provide the basis for all expected contingencies involving specific behaviours which follow from certain stimulating conditions. One might expect that an association (i.e. belief) is strengthened if an expected relationship between a particular set of stimuli and a predicted outcome is confirmed, and weakened if that outcome does not occur. However, there lies the rub because the strength of confirmation must surely be prey to how that outcome is perceived and interpreted. In a limited way this rather simplistic approach to describing a belief and how it might be acquired nonetheless serves as a model, (but by no means a scientific one) that is the premise upon which many behaviour modifying techniques and interventions are based, and described in several chapters of this book.

Let us consider the bodily sensation of pain as an example of the demonstrable power of beliefs in its persistence. Mistaken, inappropriate and unhelpful beliefs have been increasingly recognised as powerful determinants of the persistence of pain and how the affected individual adapts to it (Pincus and Morley 2002). In **Chapter 10, Burton, Waddell and Main** using an evidence-based perspective comprehensively address beliefs about back pain and provide a detailed review of recent initiatives designed specifically to target beliefs. A variety of disease processes, or some local pathology may include back pain among presenting symptoms, but back pain in the vast majority of those presenting with it is not associated with any recognisable pathology or identifiable injury and, as the authors point out, is best described as 'non-specific low back pain' or 'simple back pain' (Royal College of General Practitioners, 1999). Injury models focusing on a putative aetiological role for injury, particularly work-related injury, and progressive damage from continuing exposure to physical stressors exceeding repair, leading to disability do not explain the great majority of back pain and associated disability. Although a small proportion of people experiencing back pain will succumb to long-term incapacity the burden on health care, social security benefits, and the patients themselves is formidable.

Beliefs are moulded by experience, learning and culture, but when the development of anticipation, fears and patterns of avoidance, become established, other sources of information can play a substantial role in the formulation of beliefs about back pain. Burton, Waddell and Main highlight some beliefs about back pain with potentially detrimental characteristics that contribute to their inaccuracy. They explore the myths that represent commonly held beliefs about the nature of back pain held by the general population and the medical profession. In tackling beliefs that are obstacles to recovery/return to work the evidence suggest that appropriately focused educational interventions, across a range of environments, can change beliefs and demonstrate an accompanying effect on clinical and vocational outcomes. This approach is strongly supported by *Buchbinder (Chapter 11)*, *Horne (Chapter 8)* and *Jorm and Griffiths (Chapter 7)*. Another important message which Burton, Waddell and Main emphasize is that the development of long-term incapacity is a process in which biopsychosocial factors, separately and in combination, aggravate and perpetuate disability. The management of back pain must therefore shift from the provision of more or better health care to address these biopsychosocial factors that act as obstacles to recovery. As in other common health complaints, beliefs are important in this context and the way forward must focus on targeting inappropriate beliefs and attitudes.

One of the reasons why beliefs are important but often neglected in describing and understanding illness is that they provide a missing link between the biomedical and social systems that we as humans inhabit. Consider the fact that that despite advances in healthcare, standards of living, the absence of absolute poverty, and a consumer boom, most societies in the West are no happier than they were in the 1950's (Layard 2005). In the United Kingdom the proportion of people who are 'worried' about their health has significantly increased (Le Fanu 1999). Currently we are experiencing what can be best described as an epidemic of common health problems (worry, sadness, back pain, etc) among people in receipt of state incapacity benefits (Aylward 2004) and those who consult their general practitioners (Kroenke and Mangelsdorff 1989, Nimnuan, Hotopf *et al.* 2001, *Salmon, Chapter 9*). The great majority of people with these common health problems do not demonstrate an underlying recognisable pathological or organic basis which would account for the array and severity of the subjective complaints they report (Waddell and Burton 2004, Aylward and Sawney 2005). Moreover, even among the general population there is a surprisingly high prevalence of these common health problems (Waddell and Burton 2004), (Eriksen, Svendsrod *et al.* 1998). So what is going on? Do beliefs have any role to play here? Maybe they do. Are we seeing a manifestation of a change in individual and societal beliefs which has been brought about by the growing acceptance of a Social Theory for illness and disease? (Layard 2005, Dole and Peto 1981, McMichael 1977).

The challenge of unexplained symptoms is vigorously addressed by **Salmon in Chapter 9**. The reductionist and dualist framework which attempts to rationalize the existence of persistent medically unexplained symptoms (PMUS) comes under the hammer. Salmon argues that it is not the presence of PMUS that defines this heterogeneous group of patients; indeed symptoms of this kind are ubiquitous in the general population (Eriksen, Svendsrod *et al.* 1998, Wessely 2004) and only a proportion of 'symptomatic' people visit their doctor, most of whom do not return (Thomas 1974), or progress to disabling chronicity (Waddell and Aylward 2005). As Salmon points out, it is not the symptoms themselves but the patients' beliefs about their symptoms and what the doctor can offer that distinguish them. Moreover, Salmon provides a compelling account of the ineffectiveness of the doctors' usual responses to PMUS, illustrated by doctor-patient consultation scenarios that are ineffective, or indeed, counterproductive. Effective explanations by the doctor seem to lie at the heart of reconciling the reality of symptoms from the patient's perspective with the absence of disease. Here again the importance of effective engagement with the patient's concerns and beliefs receives substantial support (see also: Horne, Chapter 8). Of equal importance is the pivotal observation by Salmon that the clinician's failure to satisfy the patient with PMUS focuses attention on aspects of the doctor-patient interaction which are often neglected when recognisable disease is managed (see also: Jorme and Griffiths, Chapter 10).

In essence the Social Theory of illness claims that social factors associated with certain lifestyles, environmental pollutants and psychological distress are largely responsible for the upsurge in most common diseases such as cardiovascular disease and cancer, and are implicated in childhood leukaemia and the observed increase in asthma over the last 30 years or so. Undoubtedly, social and psychological factors contribute to illness and disease: lack of exercise, overindulgence in alcohol, obesity and tobacco are major challenges to public health and quite rightly, can be targeted by social interventions. Prevention of illness and disease has a compelling appeal particularly in regard to cancer and cardiovascular disease. But has the very success of this Social Theory itself changed society's own beliefs and in turn spawned a population overexposed, and excessively concerned about the ever multiplying slings and arrows of outrageous social and environmental lifestyles and toxins reported to damage health? 'Health promotion', whether as part of a benign government programme to raise awareness of unhealthy life styles and induce behaviour change, or as a consequence of a media bandwagon (which often seizes on, largely unsubstantiated 'new research which show' that some or other elements of our lifestyles or environment can be hazardous to health) can influence beliefs and behaviours. Though, one might argue, unintended, these consequences may promote unwanted preoccupation with health and are increasingly evident.

Jorm and Griffiths in Chapter 7 describe the concept of 'mental health literacy' defined as 'knowledge and beliefs about mental disorders which aid the recognition, management or prevention of these disorders' (Jorm, Korten et al. 1997). This view departs from previous thinking in this area, by emphasizing the importance of public beliefs and actions, and contrasts with the influential Pathways to Care model of Goldberg and Huxley (1992). In that model the viewpoint is very much that of the hospital-based specialist psychiatrist who asks 'How have my patients got to me?' This is a doctor-driven process which views the person with the mental health problem as largely passive; relegating the role merely to one who exhibits 'illness behaviour'.

The mental health literacy framework, however, focuses on the perspective of the person who is affected by disabling symptoms and asks, 'What can I do to feel better?' with seeking professional help being only one of a range of options. Empowering the person experiencing disabling symptoms is a critical aspect of this framework, by placing a greater emphasis on increasing the public knowledge and skills about mental health. The importance of beliefs in medicine is well illustrated by the programme of research reviewed by Jorme and Griffiths, and emphasized by Burton, Waddell and Main (Chapter 10). Notably the actions people take, including their willingness to take evidence-based treatments (see also: Horne, Chapter 10), may well represent the differences between how the public and health care professionals respectively think about treatments for mental disorders. The belief system held by these two groups thus drive difference actions, values and behaviours. Moreover, general belief systems about health are called into play by those members of the public who have no specific knowledge of mental health. Jorme and Griffiths argue that a greater willingness by the public to accept evidence-based treatments could be achieved by improving their mental health literacy. This is regarded as an important public health goal. The range of options for changing the publics' beliefs in this regard are described; not least the potential offered by the internet to dissimilate accurate up-to-date information on mental health conditions.

If one of the unintended effects of the Social Theory account has been to alter societal beliefs in a sizeable proportion of the population, this has presumably come about due to the creation of new associations in the mind. These specify a new range of possibilities that might be expected to occur if certain behaviours are performed under certain stimulating conditions. One explanation might be that the public's belief in the authority of medicine as a source of reliable knowledge and effective practice in the management of illness and disease has been eroded (Layard 2005). Expectations, (stored associations in the mind) have been modified because a set of new alternatives (generated by the Social Theory Account) have suggested a new relationship with predicted outcomes releasing the possibilities for new interpretation and behaviours. Could this also be the reason why there has been an increasing popularity of complementary and alternative medicine? Few health care professionals address the context in which health care is delivered (Di Blasi, Harkness *et al.* 2001) when treating their patients in spite of the power of the doctor-patient consultation and relationship in influencing desired outcomes. Indeed it has been argued that the power of the placebo might be exploited by facilitating the health-enhancing qualities of the context of health care (see Chapter 4).

The power of belief in medicine is no better illustrated than when the doctor's belief in his treatment and the patient's faith (belief) in his physician produce a tangible therapeutic effect. Can such a manifestation of placebo effects be other than benign? **Duncan Double in Chapter 12** sounds a note of caution: are doctors facing up to the extent to which their treatments may be placebos? He further argues that the tendency for doctors to overvalue the accuracy of their clinical diagnosis and treatment is a major determinant of the ensuing placebo effect. It is not the power of the doctor-patient consultation in influencing desired outcomes that Double challenges nor does he believe that there is obvious deceit in contemporary medicine. More particularly he focuses on medical error, the diagnostic bias which fails to take sufficient account of psychosocial factors, overmedication of symptoms and, not least, the role of expectations by doctors both in prescribing practices and in the structured assessment of medical treatments accepted as scientifically valid. Double advocates like many others in this book that the influence of the doctor-patient relationship needs to become more open and transparent, so that doctors are not deceiving their patients, nor indeed deceiving themselves.

There is convincing evidence that the reasons why millions of patients embrace complementary and alternative medicine is that they are no longer satisfied by the current practice of orthodox medicine (Furnham 2005). The undivided attention offered by practitioners in alternative medicine and the nature and style of the consultation which focuses on, and attends, to a patient's illness beliefs enhances the power of the context opening up a two-way communication, that meets the patient's expectations.

At a time when public trust in doctors and science is undoubtedly diminishing (Horton 2003), a better understanding of patients' beliefs is clearly a priority for research and clinical practice. This case is well made by **Horne (Chapter 8)** who draws much needed attention to the well-documented findings that many patients do not adhere to the medication regimens prescribed for them by their doctors. Non-adherence to treatment is nothing new: Hippocrates reminded physicians of this very problem. Though the development of effective interventions to ensure patient compliance has been a chimera, Horne sees a way forward by effectively addressing non-adherence behaviours through a modification of specific treatment beliefs held by patients. Informed adherence (Horne and Wemman 2002) based on a model of informed choice in healthcare (Michie, Dormandy *et al.* 2003) has knowledge and beliefs as its key components. A critical component of this intervention entails eliciting patients' beliefs and identifying whether pre-existing beliefs act as barriers to an unbiased interpretation of the evidence provided by the prescribing doctor. The challenge which the prescriber has to meet is to address and modify beliefs that are probably based on misconceptions or erroneous interpretation of the evidence.

Currently around 2.6 million people receive state incapacity benefit in the UK due to a health-related problem which prevents them engaging in work (Le Fanu 1999). This group largely comprises people with subjective health complaints that are commonly not supported by pathological conditions (Le Fanu 1999, Waddell and Aylward 2005). The great majority of these common health problems in this group are also prevalent among apparently healthy people (Aylward and Sawney 2005), and are usually self-limiting, and do not result in permanent impairment. Only in a very small proportion of people who report them, do they progress to longer-term ill health and incapacity for work (Nimnuan, Hotopf et al. 2001). Indeed it could be argued that these are essentially ordinary people with manageable health problems if only provided with the right opportunities, support, and encouragement. The question then is why do some people not recover as expected?

Psychological and social factors clearly aggravate and perpetuate ill health and disability (Lightman 2005, Steptoe 2005, Waddell 2002, Burton, Waddell and Main-Chapter 10). They can also act as obstacles to recovery and barriers to return to work (Nimnuan, Hotopf et al. 2001, Grove 2004). Psychological interventions addressing beliefs can improve disability in patients with low back pain (Steptoe 2005, Von Korff and Moore 2001) and have proven effective in clinical practice (Drossman 2005). There is considerable evidence to favour a bio-psycho-social approach in both understanding and helping patients with mental health problems and physical symptoms for which no explanation is apparent (Royal College of Psychiatrists 1999). Backed by this formidable array of evidence in support of the biopsychosocial approach when successfully tackling obstacles to recovery, the British Government recently endorsed a series of pilots aimed at supporting newcomers to incapacity benefits to return to work by way of a package of support which included voluntary participation in 'condition-management' programmes. These pilots very largely, focused on interventions to manage and cope better with their health problems, to modify illness behaviours and fear-avoidance beliefs, etc, on the pretext that this concerted approach would indeed prove successful as a return-to-work initiative(Le Fanu 1999). Early results of this 'Pathways to Work' initiative have been most encouraging and lend further support to behaviour change consequent upon modifying beliefs and attitudes. However the need to modify beliefs in the successful achievement of these pilots went well beyond the target population of newcomers to benefit with manageable health problems. The programme initiated by central government would not have taken place if the beliefs and attitudes of senior politicians and civil servants, the health care professions and other stakeholders within Departments of Health and the Department for Work and Pensions, and the key players in the multidisciplinary teams required to deliver the programmes, had not also undergone change. Indeed one of the most important determinants of what may prove to be the most successful psychosocial intervention in the employment sphere has been the ownership (i.e. belief in it) attributed to it by the key stakeholders and players. How did this come about?

As one of the team of civil servants who already held an abiding belief that a biopsychosocial approach promised to reap rewards in tackling barriers to (return to) work, the real challenge concerned tackling the obstacles to belief among those of influence and power. This was formidable. Politicians and Senior Departmental decision-makers have a most understandable antipathy to anything that is perceived as 'fuzzy' or based upon complex interventions or profound 'social engineering'. This is particularly so when set against a background of tight budgets, competing interests and interventions relying more on economic models than bio-psychosocial ones. So what helped bring about a change in their beliefs and attitudes? Systematic reviews of the literature, effective communication of robustly analysed evidence, identification of what best practice there was, focus groups of key opinion makers, and recognition of the benefits to the budgets that successful interventions could bring. The key elements in changing beliefs and attitudes in this context among that specific constituency depended much on a structured, robust and authoritative strategy in communicating evidence which provided compelling arguments that barriers to work resided not only in dealing with the health problem alone but more importantly tackling the personal beliefs, psychological influences and social constraints impacting on the individuals behaviour. But hard outcome indicators alone are not enough. Ideas and new concepts also played a significant role in changing attitudes and beliefs. The evidence provided the pathway towards the formulation of reasonable concepts which stimulated further ideas and new associations in the mind. There is little doubt that the evidence-based formulation of new concepts of rehabilitation for common health problems by Waddel and Burton (2004) who worked closely with our team, and adopted that convincing approach, had a very significant influence in changing the beliefs and attitudes of the key stakeholders (see Chapter 10).

In similar vein, **Buchbinder (Chapter 11)** emphasizes the potentially vital role which wide dissemination of health information plays in successfully influencing population attitudes and beliefs which inturn lead to a change in health risk behaviours. She provides compelling arguments for, and empirical findings which support, the effectiveness of a ground-breaking mass media campaign in Victoria which promoted positive beliefs about back pain, encouraged self-coping strategies and continued activity, and reduced negative beliefs about the perceived inevitable consequences of back pain among the general public. This social marketing campaign not only produced a dramatic effect in reducing disability from back pain and reliance on health care professionals for back pain care, but most likely changed physicians beliefs and attitudes towards low back pain and its management. Although, following cessation of the media campaign there had been some decay in observed positive effects, nonetheless even after 3 years, there remained a sustained positive shift in population beliefs about back pain in Victoria. What is most welcome about this highly successful public health initiative is that the sustained change in beliefs and attitudes may now represent the accepted norm which bodes well for the achievement of long-term behavioural and belief change. Furthermore, the effectiveness of the back pain media campaign has already had an important influence on further policy developments and merits serious consideration as a model approach to develop innovative approaches to other health problems which cry out for behavioural change. 'Working Backs Scotland' was launched in October 2000 (Health Education Board for Scotland and Health and Safety Executive, 2000), and the 'Welsh Backs' campaign is currently in preparation for launch in Autumn 2006. Central to the Victorian campaign, those in Scotland and Wales has been the delivery of consistent messages to those affected by back pain by all professionals and key players to help people with back pain to understand how they can best help themselves.

Buchbinder has demonstrated ways of modifying beliefs which come more by way of serendipity than design, and thus throw some light on the processes which affect belief and behaviour change? The recent education campaigns in Australia (Buckbinder, Jolley *et al.* 2001) and Scotland (Waddell 2004) which focused upon behavioural change among people with back pain disability, revealed that it may be easier to change health care professionals beliefs and behaviours by more easily changing the beliefs of their patients who in turn substantially influenced behaviour change among health care practitioners. It is clear that we have to find the right hook upon which to hang the attractive and engaging concept that disrupts stored associations and replaces them with new.

References

Aylward M (2004). Needless unemployment: the public health crisis. *What about the Workers?* K. Holland-Elliot. London, The Royal Society of Medicine Press.

Aylward M and P Sawney (2005). Support and Rehabilitation: restoring fitness for work. *Fitness for Work.* K. Palmer. London, Faculty of Occupational Medicine.

Buckbinder R, D Jolley, *et al.* (2001). 'Population based intervention to change back pain beliefs and disability: three part evaluation.' *BMJ* **322**: 1516–1520.

Di Blasi Z, E Harkness *et al.* (2001). 'Influence of context effects on health outcomes: a systemactic review.' *Lancet* **357**: 757–762.

Dole R and R Peto (1981). *The causes of cancer.* Oxford University Press.

Drossman D (2005). A case of irritable bowel syndrome that illustrates the biopsychosocial model of illness. *Biopsychosocial Medicine.* P. White. Oxford, Oxford University Press.

Eriksen H, R Svendsrod *et al.* (1998). 'Prevalence of subjective health complaints in the Nordic European countries in 1993.' *Eur J Public Health* **8**: 294–298.

Furnham A (2005). A Complementary and alternative medicine shopping for health in post-modern times. *Biopsychosocial Medicine.* P. White. Oxford, Oxford University Press.

George E (1962). *Cognition.* London, Methuen & Co Ltd.

Goldberg D and P Huxley (1992). *Common mental disorders: A bio-social model.* London and New York, Routledge.

Grove B (2004). Obstacles to solutions. *What about the Workers?* K. Holland-Elliot. London, The Royal Society of Medicine Press.

Horne R and J Wemman (2002). 'Self-regulation and self-management in asthma: Exploring the role of illness perceptions and treatment beliefs in explaining non-adherence to preventer medication 5545'. *Psychology and Health* **17**(1): 17–32.

Horton R (2003). The Dis-Eases of Medicine *in Second Opinion: Doctors, Diseases and decitions in modern medicine.* London, Granta Publications.

Jorm A, A Korten *et al.* (1997). '"Mental health literacy?": a survey of the public's ability to recognise mental disorders and their beliefs about the effectiveness of treatment.' *Medical Journal of Australia* **166**: 182–186.

Kroenke K and D Mangelsdorff (1989). 'Common symptoms in ambulatory care: incidence, evaluation, therapy and outcome.' *Am J Med* **86**: 262–266.

Layard R (2005). *Happiness.* London, Penguin/Allen Jane.

Le Fanu J (1999). *The Rise and Fall of Modern Medicine.* London, Little, Brown and Company.

Lightman S (2005). Can neurobiology explain the relationship between stress and disease? *Biopsychosocial Medicine.* P. White. Oxford, Oxford University Press.

McMichael J (1977). 'Dietetic factors in coronary disease.' *Eur Cariol* **5**: 447–452.

Michie S, E Dormandy *et al.* (2003). 'Informed choice: Understanding knowledge in the context of screening uptake.' *Patient Education and Counselling* **50**(3): 247–253.

Nimnuan C, M Hotopf *et al.* (2001). 'Medically unexplained symptoms; an epidemiological study in seven specialities.' *Pschosom Res* **51**: 361–367.

Pincus T and S Morley (2002). *Cognitive appraisal New avenues for the prevention of chronic musculoskeletal pain and disability. Pain research and clinical management.* S. Linton. Amsterdam, Elsevier. **12**: 123–141.

Practioners R. C. o. G (1999). *Clinical guidelines for the management of acute low back pain.* London, Royal College of General Practitioners.

Psychiatrists, R. C. o. P. a. (1999). *The psychological care of medical patients; A Practical guide.* London, Wiley.

Steptoe A (2005). Remediable or preventable psychological factors in the aetiology and prognosis of medical disorders. *Biopsychosocial Medicine.* P. White. Oxford, Oxford University Press.

Thomas K (1974). 'Temporarily dependent patients in general practice.' *British Medical Journal* **268**: 625–626.

Von Korff M and J Moore (2001). 'Stepped care for back pain: activating approaches for primary care.' *Ann Intern Med* **134**: 911–917.

Waddell G (2002). *Models of Disability. Using low back pain as an example.* London, The Royal Society of Medicine Press.

Waddell G and M Aylward (2005). *Scientific and Conceptual Basis of Incapacity Benefits*, The Stationary Office.

Waddell G (2004). *The Back Pain Revolution.* Edinburgh, Churchill Livingstone.

Waddell G and A Burton (2004). *Concepts of Rehabilitation for the management of common health problems.* London, The Stationary Office.

Part 1

Conceptual and psychological perspectives

Chapter 1

A cognitive neuroscience of belief

Vaughan Bell, Peter W. Halligan, and
Hadyn D. Ellis

Introduction

Belief is one of the most commonly used yet consistently unexplained aspects
of contemporary cognitive neuroscience. Bertrand Russell claimed it was 'the
central problem in the analysis of mind' (Russell, 1921, p. 231); however, few
attempts have been made to explain the psychological or neural basis of belief
itself. This continues to be the case despite the fact that beliefs forms a central
part of our folk psychological explanations for behaviour. Unlike most other
areas of cognitive science (e.g. attention, memory, perception, language, and
action systems) cognitive neuroscience has typically neglected formal
discussion of belief. This is due to several reasons, not least the nebulous and
ill-defined nature of the construct. While free will appear to be less trouble-
some for current neuropsychology enquiry (Zhu, 2004), one might be forgiven
for asking exactly what is so difficult about belief?

Difficulties in conceptualizing the nature of belief

Agreement on a formal definition is one of the most hotly debated issues in
contemporary philosophy and has obvious implications for any cognitive
neuropsychological approach to belief.

The simple statement 'I believe that . . . ' belies a large number of possible
interpretations of what is actually happening in the human brain when
someone makes such a claim. One of the most remarkable things about belief
is the ease and acceptance of such straight-forward statements in everyday life
without. While the number of possible interpretations may cause surprisingly
little distraction for the casual listener, it causes a great deal of consternation
for the cognitive scientist who needs to define the processes involved to be able
to understand how it may operate and be supported by the neural systems of
the brain.

The issue at stake here, however, is not whether we find the concept of belief useful in everyday communication, but whether this everyday understanding of belief is valid such that it can be used for scientific investigation and, in particular, for those seeking to link the construct to selective cognitive process and their underlying neural states. The problem is more widely discussed among philosophers of mind (the philosophical study of the nature of the mental events) rather than cognitive scientists. Moreover, it is often difficult to make a clear distinction between questions of whether a neuropsychology of belief is possible, and what the likely nature of that belief might be. Although conceptually distinct, in practice, the latter tends to have considerable implications for the former. Baker (1987) identifies four major views on the 'correctness' of the everyday understanding of belief and how it may relate to underlying neural processes:

1 **Our common-sense understanding of belief is correct.** The common-sense view of belief (i.e. folk belief) tends to equate beliefs with explicitly held propositions. Here, such propositions are available as representations in memory and consulted when an appropriate situation arises. Among philosophers who have argued for beliefs as representations, Fodor (1975) is a particularly well-known exponent. Controversially, he has argued that a fundamental 'language of thought' – independent of the actual spoken language of the believer – underlies the representation of belief (and other mental states). A discussion of his 'language of thought' hypothesis is outside the scope of this chapter; however, this syntactic description of belief is not without its critics, and the strength of the passion it engenders can be seen from a repost by Still and Costall who went as far as to describe Fodor's theories as 'where one tries to keep a reasonably straight face while presenting the absurd consequences of the scheme as exciting theoretical revelations' (Still and Costall, 1991, p. 2).

The belief as representation' hypothesis, however, does not necessarily entail subscribing to an underlying language of thought. Both Armstrong (1973) and Dretske (1988) have argued that beliefs may be stored as semantic maps, an idea which seems a good deal less speculative now – in the light of recent advances in understanding how neural systems might encode even high-level information topographically or in multidimensional arrays (Lloyd, 2000, 2002) – than it may have seemed when first introduced.

2 **Our common-sense understanding of belief may not be entirely correct, but it is close enough to make some useful predictions.** This view argues that we will eventually reject the construct of belief as we now use it, but that there may be a correlation between what we take to be a belief when

someone says 'I believe that snow is white' and how a future theory of psychology will explain this behaviour. In a way, this is a 'missing link' argument which suggests that we talk about circumscribed beliefs and particular brain states, but are missing an important conceptual link which will change our understanding of how the two are connected and will cause us to rethink our model of belief (or even eliminate it). We can perhaps draw an analogy between how we now understand hemispatial neglect in terms of an attentional deficit to one side of space and how, through the ages, the same behaviour was undoubtedly explained as sensory loss. The traditional explanation may be no longer sustainable under rigorous scientific investigation, but some of the practical implications may be similar. Most notably, Stich (1983) has argued for this particular understanding of belief with his 'panglossian' approach.

3 **Our common-sense understanding of belief is entirely wrong and will be completely superseded by a radically different theory which will have no use for the concept of belief as we know it.** Known as eliminative materialism or eliminativism, this view, most notably proposed by Churchland (1981, 1999), argues that the concept of belief is like other old, obsolete theories, such as the four humours theory of medicine or the phlogiston theory of combustion. In these cases science has not provided us with a more detailed account of these theories, but completely rejected them as valid scientific concepts to be replaced by entirely different accounts. Churchland argues that our common-sense concept of belief is similar, in that, as we discover more about neuroscience and the brain, the inevitable conclusion will be to reject the belief hypothesis in its entirety. Although Churchland may make bleak reading for anyone wishing to retain the concept of belief in any sort of explanatory framework, one implication of this view is that our current concept of belief will be replaced by a number of better specified neuropsychological theories.

4 **Our common-sense understanding of belief is entirely wrong. However, treating people, animals, and even computers as if they had beliefs is often a successful and pragmatic strategy.** Dennett (1999) and Baker (1987) are both eliminativists in that they argue that beliefs are not adequately reducible to their neural underpinnings, but they do not go as far as rejecting the concept of belief as a predictive device. Baker (1987, p. 150) gives the example of playing a computer at chess. While few people would agree that the computer held beliefs, treating the computer as if it did (e.g. that the computer believes that taking the opposition's queen will give it a considerable advantage) is likely to be a successful and predictive strategy. In this understanding of belief, called 'interpretationism', or, in Dennett's terminology

taking the 'the intentional stance', belief-based explanations of mind and behaviour provide a convenient level of explanation and, while not ultimately reducible (unlike other cognitive constructs such as memory), could be of explanatory value in itself.

Others have similarly suggested that beliefs are best understood as 'dispositions to act' in a certain way in certain circumstances, and argue against the common-sense, representational view of belief, given the implausibility of its consequences. If you were asked 'do you believe tigers wear pink pyjamas?', you would say you do not, despite the fact that you may have never thought about this situation before. You are also likely to believe that there are fewer than three people in a duet, as well as believing that there are fewer than four people in a duet, fewer than five . . . and so on, *ad infinitum*. Proponents of the dispositional view of belief (such as Marcus, 1990) claim that such examples show that beliefs cannot simply be representations of 'facts' in the brain, as it would be impossible to have an infinite number of beliefs stored in finite neural structures. They claim that beliefs are therefore dispositional and only ascribable to observable behaviour in others.

Initially, this seems like a behaviourist approach to belief, and, unsurprisingly, was initially championed by philosophers such as Gilbert Ryle (1949), who were sympathetic to many of the goals of behaviourist psychology. Others (such as Schwitzgebel, 2002) have argued for a more liberal and less strictly behaviourist interpretation of the dispositional account, where dispositions could include non-observable behaviour and responses, such as emotional reactions or cognitive reorganization. This approach also suggests that our current conception of belief is realized as multiple neuropsychological systems.

Are beliefs discrete entities?

The views expressed above can be thought of as discussions regarding the fundamental nature of belief and/or its dependency, or not, on neural systems. A further issue concerns whether it makes sense to conceive of beliefs (whatever their structure) as independent entities (i.e. circumscribed psychological units or cognitive systems), or whether beliefs only exist as coherent entities when conceptualized as part of a wider network of beliefs. The former position is known as atomism, the latter holism, and the distinction becomes clear when issues arise as to whether the same beliefs can be considered identical for any given referent. For example Price (1934, 1969), an atomist, conceived of beliefs as single propositions; so two people would be considered to hold the same belief if they both assent to the same belief sentence (e.g. 'snow is white'). Alternatively, proponents of the holist view (Davidson, 1973, 1984; Quine and Ullian, 1970) argued that beliefs can only be understood in terms of their relation to other beliefs. For example if two people express the belief that 'snow is white' but one believes it is made of star-dust while the other believes it is frozen water, a holist would argue that they are not expressing the same belief, as they have radically different conceptions about the nature of snow.

This distinction is important for neuropsychologists, because it potentially defines the link between belief claims and how they relate to the underlying neuropsychological processes which support them. For example an atomist would expect that similar neural activation would occur for an identical task that relied on the same belief that p, regardless of whether additional beliefs relating to p are accepted or rejected over time. In contrast, a holist might expect brain activity to be radically different if and when new beliefs relating to p are acquired, as p can only be understood in the context of its interconnectedness with other beliefs. Therefore, a holist view is more likely to support a multifactorial neuropsychological account of belief, as multiple processes or multiple sites of neural activation might be involved by nature of the fact that then activation of any particular belief would involve the activation of related beliefs. This tradition might see belief as simply a linguistic label for a number of disparate cognitive processes, suggesting that the neural underpinnings of what we understand someone to be doing when they say 'I believe that . . . ' to be many and various and best explained as a complex system of more fundamental neuropsychological processes (Horgan and Woodward, 1985).

The dominant theme that arises from these philosophical perspectives is that there is unlikely to be a unitary belief formation process explained by a monolithic neuropsychological model. As such competing theories can be seen as making predictions about the likely neural involvement in belief processing, these can be compared with experimental data to provide evidence for the ongoing debate in the philosophy of mind. However, in the next section, the focus moves from philosophy of mind to consider how current clinical and theoretical based neuroscience approaches have contributed to understanding the nature of belief.

Cognitive neuroscience approaches

Given that 'theories in the cognitive sciences are largely about the belief organisms have' (Fodor, 1981), one might expect considerable interest within the cognitive neuroscience community. The case for a neuropsychological basis for belief has received some debate in the neuroscience literature; however, most do not explicitly address beliefs as a discrete mental category but rather concern the relationship of mind to biological function. Moreover, most accounts do not distinguish between beliefs as a neurological phenomenon (based entirely on the biology of the brain), and neuropsychological explanations, based on information-processing or functional approaches models of assumed underlying neural function. The paucity of studies reflect some of the problems outlined earlier regarding the philosophical nature and definition of belief.

Until recently the explicit study of beliefs has not attracted particular interest, with the exception of research into 'theory of mind' (the theorized ability to represent another person's beliefs and intentions). Indeed, 'theory of mind' ('mind reading') is often described in terms of belief (or false belief), yet it is not clear how explicitly current studies tackle the base construct. As Dennett (1978) has noted, in many instances predicting others' behaviour can be done without a 'theory of mind' and can be completed simply by observing the actual state of the world. Similarly, the relationship between the false belief task and 'theory of mind' is unclear, despite the fact that many studies conflate the two (Bloom and German, 2000), making 'theory of mind' research a potentially poor candidate on which to base any general theories of belief.

One novel and ingenious approach has been taken recently by Goel and Dolan (2003) who conducted an fMRI study using Evans, Handley, and Harper's (2001) belief-modulated reasoning paradigm. Evans' group found that syllogistic reasoning is impaired when the outcome of a problem is in conflict with an individual's belief, despite being correct in the context of the presented problem (e.g. no addictive things are inexpensive; some cigarettes are inexpensive; therefore some cigarettes are not addictive). Goel and Dolan compared brain activation between syllogisms where the correct answer was in agreement with the participants' beliefs, those that were belief discordant, and a condition using non-belief reasoning (e.g. all A are B; all B are C; therefore all A are C) to elicit activation specifically related to the effect of belief on reasoning. They reported left temporal activation for belief-based reasoning, and ventral medial prefrontal cortex activation when pre-existing beliefs caused reasoning to go awry, whereas successful suppression of belief for successful reasoning was associated with right lateral prefrontal activation. They concluded that belief-bias effects in reasoning may affect reasoning through emotional processing mechanisms known to involve the medial ventral prefrontal cortex, a conclusion not unrelated to much of Frijda's work on the links between emotion and belief (Frijda et al., 2000).

While Goel and Dolan's study remains neutral with regard to a specific philosophical theory of belief (belief as representation, disposition, etc.), a study by Gallagher et al. (2002) specifically tackles belief by attempting to image the 'intentional stance' (Dennett, 1999) – the predictive strategy whereby we interpret the behaviour of another by assuming a rational agent whose behaviour is governed by intentional states. In this study, participants were asked to play the game 'paper, scissors, stone' against an opponent whose responses were displayed on a computer screen. In one condition participants were told that they were playing against a human opponent, in the other the responses were randomly generated by a computer. In fact, in both conditions the responses were randomly generated, but when participants believed they were playing against a human there was significantly greater bilateral anterior paracingulate activation, which, the researchers suggest, shows a specific neural response for taking the 'intentional stance'. Although the findings of Gallagher *et al.* (2002) are of interest, it is not clear how useful they are for understanding the functional anatomy of beliefs unless one assumes that our ability to explain and predict other people's behaviour (i.e. 'theory of mind'), by attributing mental states and/or by taking an 'intentional stance', is operationally equivalent to adopting or holding a specific belief.

Neuropsychological correlates of paranormal beliefs

One aspect of the study of beliefs that has attracted disproportionate attention is belief in the paranormal, not least because of its potential links with religion and psychosis (Persinger and Makarec, 1990; Peters, 2001). Paranormal belief has also been particularly linked to increased right hemisphere activation, and a reduction in left hemisphere dominance for language. Whilst Crow (1997) has controversially argued that this pattern is associated with the expression of frank psychosis and schizophrenia, it is certainly clear that this activation asymmetry is also associated with paranormal beliefs that are not accompanied by a psychiatric diagnosis. It has been reported that a belief in extra-sensory perception (ESP) in non-patients is associated with increased right hemisphere activation (Brugger *et al.*, 1993a, 1993b), a finding which has also been replicated with measures of paranormal belief and neuropsychological measures such as of electroencephalography (EEG) (Pizzagalli *et al.*, 2000), olfactory discrimination (Mohr *et al.*, 2001), and line bisection (Taylor *et al.*, 2002).

Leonhard and Brugger (1998) argue that this lateralized pattern signifies over-reliance on right hemisphere processes, whose coarse rather than focused semantic processing may favour the emergence of 'loose' and 'uncommon' associations. They consider these effects lying on a continuum, whereby in some they contribute to novel thought and creativity and in other psychosis. However, it is unlikely that the degree of medically diagnosable 'illness' is a simple correlation with degree of hemispheric asymmetry, as many other factors (such as sociocultural factors, individual history, and coping styles) also contribute to such cognitive influences, beliefs and experiences being impairing, distressing, or disabling rather than considered as normal belief (Bentall, 2003).

Reports of hemispheric asymmetries and paranormal belief have also been described by Persinger (1983), who has amassed considerable converging evidence suggesting that right temporal lobe activity is associated with paranormal belief (the term 'paranormal' is used here in its widest sense, also to include religious and mystical beliefs). Persinger (1983) argues that mystical experience and religious beliefs are the normal consequence of transient activity in the tempero-limbic structures and has subsequently found that the strength of paranormal beliefs was positively correlated with the amount of activation in these structures. This correlation was found in individuals engaged in psychic studies (Persinger and Fisher, 1990), during specific episodes of glossolalia ('speak in tongues'), and transcendental meditation (Persinger, 1984) and with more general measure of paranormal experience (Persinger and Valliant, 1985).

The main implication of these neuropsychological findings is that widely-held religious, mystical, or paranormal beliefs are associated with specific patterns of cortical and subcortical activation. These can be studied by developing standardized psychometric questionnaires that can be the basis of drawing neuropsychological inference, as long as they are well validated by the appropriate application of cognitive neuroscience.

Delusions as false beliefs

If the underlying cognitive (and by extension neural architecture) for belief and belief formation was organized as a modular system, then the study of brain injury (or the application of other module-friendly experimental methods) could provide (depending on location and combination) another production line of empirical investigation. The lesion method has proved to be a powerful tool for cognitive neuropsychologists in charting the potential relationship between mind and brain. Indeed, some forms of cognitive neuropsychology are only viable if the hypothetical modules envisaged in mind are both conceptually distinct in terms of the overall cognitive system and spatially distinct in terms of their putative anatomical location (Shallice, 1988). Brain injury may selectively damage cognitive modules, so their existence and function may be inferred from the experience, abilities, and behaviour of postinjury patients (Shallice, 1988).

Notwithstanding Fodor's prediction that beliefs, as highly elaborate knowledge systems, are the product of 'central' rather than modular processes (Fodor, 2000), there are useful parallels to be drawn between the successful and ongoing research into the executive system and attempts to understand the neuropsychology of belief (Bell et al., 2003a). Drawing inspiration from

Burgess' (1997) analysis of methodology in executive function research, Bell *et al.* (2003) note that the executive system as currently understood fulfils many of Fodor's criteria for a 'central' process. Burgess argues that there is no direct 'process–behaviour correspondence', so that the executive system can only be seen to be working indirectly through the measurement of other cognitive processes with which it integrates. If belief is indeed a central process it may well operate in a similar manner and, as such, any attempts to find a single point of measurement (or single point of breakdown) would be inappropriate.

Given the caution Burgess points out with regard to employing and relying on single probes for complex interacting psychological constructs, it may seem strange that one avenue which has proved productive in the understanding of beliefs has been the study of delusions (i.e. 'pathologies of belief'). The recent application of a cognitive neuropsychology approaches to psychiatric symptoms (cognitive neuropsychiatry) attempts to better understand normal psychological function by studying psychopathology and by explaining psychiatric symptoms in terms of normal models of neuropsychological function (David and Halligan, 1996; Halligan and David, 2001). Early successes have produced specific and plausible mechanisms for how certain pathological beliefs might arise, most notably for the Capgras delusion (Breen *et al.*, 2000; Ellis and Young, 1990; Ellis and Lewis, 2001; Hirstein and Ramachandran, 1997). In this account, damage to an unconscious face recognition pathway is impaired, leaving Capgras sufferers without the appropriate emotional response to familiar faces, potentially explaining why they may come to believe familiar people have been replaced by identical-looking impostors.

Unlike physical lesions or specific perceptual-based disturbances, delusions are not as easily quantified or defined. Despite being typically treated as pathological versions of normal belief formation, it has become increasingly clear that delusions are far more complex than originally represented in traditional psychiatry (Bell *et al.*, 2003a; David, 1999).

Although it is by no means clear, converging methods currently employed by neuroscience could provide the conceptual glue that may eventually bind the physical and psychological levels of explanation with regard to the 'problem of belief'. The three approaches discussed above (functional neuroimaging, the lesion method, and examining neurophysiological and neuropsychological correlates of belief states) all provide valid approaches to the neuropsychology of belief. However, what is equally important is formulating a well-specified, conceptually constrained model to help guide and direct all three approaches.

A model for belief formation

Belief formation is a complex process and, as already noted in the philosophy of mind literature, is likely to be supported by a number of processes. Bentall (1990) produced a simple conceptual cyclic model (Fig. 1.1) which seems to capture some intuitive aspects of belief formation; however, there are several reasons why this model is inadequate.

1 Philosophers and common sense argued that we do not choose our beliefs (review in Engel, 2002). For example we cannot decide to believe that it is snowing in Devon unless we have evidence that it is – or more obviously, disbelieve it is raining if we are getting rained on. This suggests that an adequate model of belief formation must involve both an explicitly unconscious component, as well as a process of conscious evaluation.

2 One aspect which seems particularly important is the role of the 'web of belief' in the belief formation process. This seems a necessary condition for beliefs to be meaningful, as well as an important process in the acceptance, rejection, assimilation, and integration of beliefs. Quine and Ullian (1970) noted beliefs must be integrated into our current web of belief, which may itself be changed (for example some beliefs may be mutually exclusive) as new beliefs are added. Indeed, the need to account for a 'web of beliefs' in belief formation processes has long been recognized. Davidson (1973, 1984) has been an influential proponent of the view that beliefs can only be understood by relating them to a background of other beliefs and desires; Fodor (1978) draws the conclusions from his 'language of thought' hypothesis that beliefs must necessarily be related to and justified by reference to other propositions. In social psychology, theories of belief networks are central to many theories on the psychology of attitudes (Eagly and Chaiken, 1993). Cognitive dissonance theory, as first proposed by Festinger (1957), has the discrepancy between active beliefs as eliciting a drive to make them coherent, and even many of the reinterpretations are essentially belief coherence

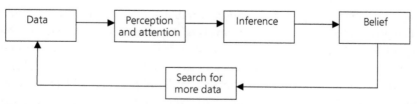

Fig. 1.1 Bentall's (1990) 'back of an envelope' model of belief formation.

models (Harman-Jones and Mills, 2002). Similarly, cognitive balance theory, another foundational model in social psychology, has attitudes and beliefs as necessarily existing in relation to other attitudes (Heider, 1946; Abelson, 1986).

Indeed, even despite the relative paucity of neuropsychological models of belief formation, this integrative process is crucial. Stone and Young's (1997) strongly argue that belief formation involves weighing up explanations that are observationally adequate versus those that fit within a person's current belief set. 'Observationally adequate' could be interpreted here in a number of ways. For example work by Maio (2002), who has studied the belief in social values such as freedom and equality, found that the number of reasons people produced by to support these beliefs is typically less than other beliefs. This suggests that some important beliefs may not be so highly interconnected, or, at least, such connections are not always available to consciousness or easy to articulate.

3 This suggests an important role for emotion in belief formation, a view which has not been without support. (Fridja *et al.*, 2000; Evans and Cruse, 2004). Social psychological research is now increasingly defining 'attitudes' in terms of both cognitive and affective components and propensities of individuals preferentially to favour these components in forming attitudes (Haddock and Zanna, 2000). Therefore, the influence of emotion on belief must be included in any complete model of belief formation.

4 Beliefs exist with differing degrees of confidence as to their likelihood or validity. A belief formation model should not simply 'output' a belief as having been accepted or rejected, but allow for a degree of conviction in the belief statement. Although there is reason to think that, ultimately, this may not break down into a simple, single dimension of belief (Harman, 1988, for example, has convincingly argued that, in some cases, people may be justified in having a higher degree of confidence in a proposition in which they do not believe than in a proposition that they do believe), a tacit acknowledgement that beliefs are not 'all-or-nothing' entities would seem to be essential to give any successful model of belief face validity.

5 Finally, beliefs may also formed on the basis of testimony rather than direct experience, a type of belief Rokeach (1968) called authority beliefs. An acceptable theory of belief must include the ability to hold these sort of 'second hand' beliefs, without direct perceptual experience of the subject of the belief.

A candidate neuropsychological model of belief formation

While models of belief formation have been specified before in psychology, these have typically been created on a common-sense view of belief, without any regard to neuropsychological mechanisms which might support the process, or whether they are coherent in terms of their relation to supporting neurological structures. There is currently a paucity of explicitly neuropsychological models of belief formation, although a candidate model is reviewed below.

Possibly the most explicitly-specified model, derived from a cognitive neuropsychiatric analysis of delusions, is from Langdon and Coltheart (2000). As can be seen from Fig. 1.2, their model takes a three-stage approach: the first stage consists of monitoring processes that alert an individual to information in the environment, which may be novel or personally relevant. The second stage concerns the generation of hypotheses to explain any information that might be made salient by the earlier monitoring stage; with the final stage involving the evaluation of all possible explanations, a process by which the

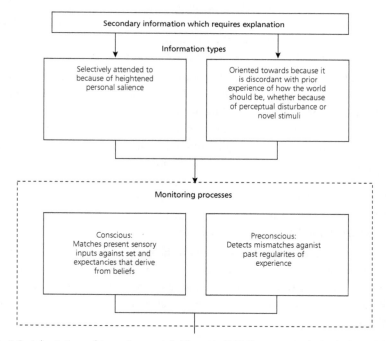

Fig. 1.2 Adaptation of Langdon and Coltheart's (2000) neuropsychological model of belief formation.

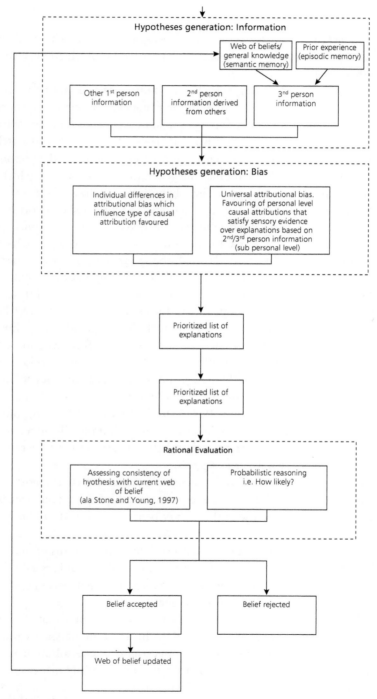

Fig. 1.2 (*Cont.*)

most rational (or most likely) explanation is accepted as a belief. The monitoring stage acts as a filtering system to decide which sensory information is worthy of further consideration.

Langdon and Coltheart specify both a conscious and an unconscious component to this stage, including in their model a conscious monitoring process that matches sensory inputs against expectancies that derive from beliefs and an unconscious monitoring process that detects mismatches against past regularities of experience. Information that passes the presumed salience threshold might then cause the generation of hypotheses, which, in turn, may explain the experience. These hypotheses are drawn from a variety of information sources, including first-, second-, and third-person information, as well as episodic memory and a pre-existing 'web of beliefs' (drawing in part from semantic memory). It is at this stage that the hypotheses are weighted to enable a prioritized 'list' to be formed, the weightings being assigned by various sources of bias. Langdon and Coltheart argue that these may stem from either one of two sources. Their first source is universal influences (although we may be a little suspicious of the use of the term 'universal' here, and most people will probably be happier with the less grand 'sociocultural') such as the favouring of personal over subpersonal level explanations. The other is individual differences in attributional biases, such as those identified by Bentall *et al.* (1991) in pathological states (such as a tendency to blame negative events on others), or non-pathological biases that may occur in everyday life (Graham and Folkes, 1990; Mezulis *et al.*, 2004). These hypotheses are then subjected to rational evaluation where both probabilistic reasoning and agreement with the current 'web of belief' is used either to accept the belief (and update the web) or to reject it.

Langdon and Coltheart's is a useful working model that covers most of the criteria referred to earlier for an adequate model. Some crucial processes however, particularly the use of the 'web of belief' to assimilate and test new beliefs, are left as theoretical black boxes. As discussed earlier, this may be an essential part of any model of belief; potentially both in terms of making a pretheoretical concept of belief coherent (as the holists would argue) and/or to capture the empirical data concerning the interconnectedness of beliefs and the influence of other beliefs on belief formation.

Similarly, perhaps we have to be a little generous in assuming that emotional effects on belief are adequately explained by the 'attributional biases' process of this model. Whilst affective factors almost certainly alter attribution, relying purely on the cognitive neuropsychiatric approach unduly dispenses with much good work done on normal belief in this area (see the aforementioned Frijda *et al.*, 2000).

Conclusions

One important conclusion from this comparison is that a cognitive neuro-psychiatric approach to belief may lead to useful developments and testable theories. As the only explicitly neuropsychological model of belief of its type, Langdon and Coltheart's (2000) model is remarkably well specified, despite some notable ambiguities in their explanation of the operation of the component processes. However, these current models further suggest that the study of delusions, belief pathology, and even simply 'anomalous' belief is likely to be a useful and productive approach to understanding normal belief.

References

Abelson RP (1986). Beliefs and like possessions. *Journal for the Theory of Behaviour*, **16**, 223–250.

Armstrong, DM (1973). *Belief, truth, and knowledge*. Cambridge: Cambridge University Press.

Baker LR (1987). *Saving belief: a critique of physicalism*. Princeton: Princeton University Press.

Bell V, Ellis H and Halligan P (2003a). Neuropsychology, delusions and modularity: The curious problem of belief. *Proceedings of the British Psychological Society*, **11**, 174.

Bell V, Halligan PW and Ellis H (2003b). Beliefs about delusions. *Psychologist*, **16**, 418–423.

Bentall R (2003). *Madness explained: psychosis and human nature*. London: Penguin Books.

Bentall RP (ed) (1990). *Reconstructing Schizophrenia*. London: Routledge, pp. 23–60.

Bentall RP, Kaney S and Dewey ME (1991). Paranoia and social reasoning: An attribution theory analysis. *British Journal of Clinical Psychology*, **31**, 12–23.

Bloom P and German TP (2000). Two reasons to abandon the false belief task as a test of theory of mind. *Cognition*, **77**, 25–31.

Breen N, Caine C, Coltheart M, Hendy J and Roberts C (2000). Towards and understanding of delusions of misidentification. In: M Coltheart and M Davies, eds. *Pathologies of belief*. Oxford: Blackwell.

Brugger P, Gamma A, Muri R, Schafer M and Taylor KI (1993a). Functional hemispheric asymmetry and belief in ESP: towards a 'neuropsychology of belief'. *Perceptual and Motor Skills*, **77**, 1299–1308.

Brugger P, Regard M, Landis T, Cook N, Krebs D and Niederberger J (1993b). 'Meaningful' patterns in visual noise: effects of lateral stimulation and the observer's belief in ESP. *Psychopathology*, **26**, 261–265.

Burgess PW (1997). Theory and methodology in executive function research. In: P Rabbitt, ed. *Methodology of frontal and executive function*, pp. 81–116. Hove: Psychology Press.

Churchland P (1981). Eliminative materialism and the propositional attitudes. *Journal of Philosophy*, **78**, 67–90.

Churchland P (1999). Current eliminativism. In: W Lycan, ed. *Mind and cognition*, 2nd edn. Oxford: Blackwell.

Crow TJ (1997). Schizophrenia as failure of hemispheric dominance for language. *Trends in Neurosciences*, **20**, 339–343.

David AS (1999). On the impossibility of defining delusions. *Philosophy, Psychiatry, and Psychology*, **6**, 17–20.

David AS and Halligan PW (1996). Editorial. *Cognitive Neuropsychiatry*, 1, 1–3.

Davidson D (1973). Radical interpretation. *Dialectica*, **27**, 313–328.

Davidson D (1984). *Inquiries into truth and interpretation*. Oxford: Clarendon.

Dennett D (1978). Beliefs about beliefs. *Behavioral and Brain Sciences*, **1**, 568–570.

Dennett D (1999). An instrumentalist theory. True believers: The intentional strategy and why it works. In: W Lycan, ed. *Mind and cognition*, 2nd edn. Oxford: Blackwell.

Dretske F (1988). *Explaining behavior: Reasons in a world of causes*. London: MIT Press.

Eagly A and Chaiken S (1993). *The psychology of attitudes*. Orlando: Harcourt Brace and Company.

Ellis HD and Lewis MB (2001). Capgras delusion: a window on face recognition. *Trends in Cognitive Sciences*, **5**, 149–156.

Ellis HD and Young AW (1990). Accounting for delusional misidentifications. *British Journal of Psychiatry*, **157**, 239–248.

Engel P (2002). Free believers. In: J Pessoa, A Leclerc, G da Silva de Queiroz and MB Wrigley, eds. *Manuscrito*, vol. 15 (Special Number, Mental Causation). Proceedings of the Third International Colloquium in Philosophy of Mind, Brazil: Unicamp. pp. 155–175.

Evans D and Cruse P (2004). *Emotion, evolution and rationality*. Oxford: Oxford University Press.

Evans JS, Handley SJ and Harper CN (2001). Necessity, possibility and belief: a study of syllogistic reasoning. *Quarterly Journal of Experimental Psychology A*, **54**, 935–958.

Festinger L (1957). *A theory of cognitive dissonance*. Stanford: Stanford University Press.

Fodor J (1975). *The language of thought*. New York: Crowell.

Fodor J (1978). Propositional attitudes. *Monist*, **61**, 501–523.

Fodor J (1981). The mind-body problem. *Scientific American*, **244**, 114–123.

Fodor J (2000). *The mind doesn't work that way: the scope and limits of computational biology*. Cambridge, MA: MIT Press.

Frijda NH, Manstead ASR and Bem S (2000). *Emotions and beliefs: How feelings influence thoughts*. Cambridge: Cambridge University Press.

Gallagher HL, Jack AI, Roepstroff A and Frith CD (2002). Imaging the intentional stance in a competitive game. *Neuroimage*, **16**, 814–821.

Goel V and Dolan RJ (2003). Explaining modulation of reasoning by belief. *Cognition*, **87**, B11–B22.

Graham S and Folkes VS (1990). *Attributions to achievement, mental health and interpersonal conflict*. Hillsdale, NJ: Lawrence Erlbaum Associates.

Haddock G and Zanna MP (2000). Cognition, affect, and the prediction of social attitudes. In: W Stroebe and M Hewstone, eds. *European review of social psychology*. Chichester, England: Wiley.

Halligan PW and David AS (2001). Cognitive neuropsychiatry: Towards a scientific psychopathology. *Nature Neuroscience Review*, **2**, 209–215.

Harman G (1988). *Change in view: principles of reasoning*. London: Bradford Books.

Harman-Jones E and Mills J (2002). An introduction to cognitive dissonance theory and an overview of current perspectives on the theory. In: E Harman-Jones and J Mills, eds.

Cognitive dissonance: progress on a pivotal theory in cognitive psychology. Washington: American Psychological Association.

Heider, F (1946). Attitudes and cognitive organization. *The Journal of Psychology*, **21**, 107–112.

Hirstein W and Ramachandran VS (1997). Capgras syndrome: a novel probe for understanding the neural representation of the identity and familiarity of persons. *Proceedings of the Royal Society of London B: Biological Sciences*, **264**, 437–444.

Horgan T and Woodward J (1985). Folk psychology is here to stay. *Philosophical Review*, **94**, 197–226.

Langdon R and Coltheart M (2000). The cognitive neuropsychology of delusions. In: M Coltheart and M Davies, eds. *Pathologies of belief*. Oxford: Blackwell. 183–216.

Leonhard D and Brugger P (1998). Creative, paranormal, and delusional thought: a consequence of right hemisphere semantic activation? *Neuropsychiatry, Neuropsychology and Behavioral Neurology*, **11**, 177–183.

Lloyd D (2000). Terra cognita: from functional neuroimaging to the map of the mind. *Brain and Mind*, **1**, 1–24.

Lloyd D (2002). Functional MRI and the study of human consciousness. *Journal of Cognitive Neuroscience*, **14**, 818–831.

Maio GR (2002). Values-Truth and meaning. *The Psychologist*, **15**, 296–299.

Marcus RB (1990). Some revisionary proposals about belief and believing. *Philosophy and Phenomenological Research*, **50**, 132–153.

Mezulis AH, Abramson LY, Hyde JS and Hankin BL (2004). Is there a universal positivity bias in attributions?: A meta-analytic review of individual, developmental, and cultural differences in the self-serving attributional bias. *Psychological Bulletin*, **130**, 711–747.

Mohr C, Rohrenbach CM, Laska M and Brugger P (2001). Unilateral olfactory perception and magical ideation. *Schizophrenia Research*, **47**, 255–264.

Persinger MA (1983). Religious and mystical experiences as artifacts of temporal lobe function: a general hypothesis. *Perceptual and Motor Skills*, **57**, 1255–1262.

Persinger MA (1984). Striking EEG profiles from single episodes of glossolalia and transcendental meditation. *Perceptual and Motor Skills*, **58**, 127–133.

Persinger MA and Fisher SD (1990). Elevated, specific temporal lobe signs in a population engaged in psychic studies. *Perceptual and Motor Skills*, **71**, 817–818.

Persinger MA and Makarec K (1990). Exotic beliefs may be substitutes for religious beliefs. *Perceptual and Motor Skills*, **71**, 16–18.

Persinger MA and Valliant PM (1985). Temporal lobe signs and reports of subjective paranormal experiences in a normal population: a replication. *Perceptual and Motor Skills*, **60**, 903–909.

Peters E (2001). Are delusions on a continuum ? The case of religious and delusional beliefs. In: I Clarke, ed. *Psychosis and spirituality: exploring the new frontier*. London: Whurr Publishers.

Pizzagalli D, Lehmann D, Gianotti L, Koenig T, Tanaka H, Wackermann J, *et al.* (2000). Brain electric correlates of strong belief in paranormal phenomena: intracerebral EEG source and regional Omega complexity analyses. *Psychiatry Research*, **100**, 139–154.

Price HH (1934). Some considerations about belief. *Proceedings of the Aristotelian Society*, **35**, 229–252.

Price HH (1969). *Belief.* London: Allen and Unwin.

Quine WV and Ullian JS (1970). *The web of belief.* New York: Random House.

Rokeach M (1968). *Beliefs, attitudes and values: a theory of organization and change.* San Francisco: Jossey-Bass.

Russell B (1921). *The analysis of mind.* New York: McMillan.

Ryle G (1949). *The concept of mind.* New York: Barnes and Noble.

Schwitzgebel E (2002). A phenomenal, dispositional account of belief. *Nous,* **36**, 249–275.

Shallice T (1988). *From neuropsychology to mental structure.* Cambridge: Cambridge University Press.

Stich S (1983). *From folk psychology to cognitive science: the case against belief.* Cambridge, MA: MIT Press.

Still A and Costall A, eds (1991). *Against cognitivism: alternative foundations for cognitive psychology.* London: Harvester Wheatsheaf.

Stone, T and Young AW (1997). Delusions and brain injury: The philosophy and psychology of belief. *Mind and Language,* **12**, 327–364.

Taylor KI, Zach P, *et al.* (2002). Why is magical ideation related to leftward deviation on an implicit line bisection task? *Cortex,* **38**, 247–252.

Zhu J (2004). Understanding volition. *Philosophical Psychology,* **17**, 247–273.

Chapter 2

Biased beliefs and the subjective validation effect

David F. Marks

Introduction

In this chapter, I describe some recent research on biased beliefs and the phenomenon of 'subjective validation'. Subjective validation occurs when a person maintains her/his prior beliefs when given clear and unambiguous evidence to the contrary. There are reasons to believe that the subjective validation effect is quite a common, if not a universal, phenomenon in human reasoning and judgement.

When we consider the more bizarre beliefs, such as those that relate to the paranormal, there is new evidence that the subjective validation effect is associated with schizotypy, fantasy proneness, and vividness of imagery. It is predicted that subjective validation will be moderated by a person's level of schizotypy, such that high schizotypes will maintain their prior beliefs in psi significantly longer than low schizotypes when given evidence to the contrary. The relationships between the characteristics of fantasy proneness, imagery vividness, and transliminality with subjective validation, paranormal beliefs, and schizotypy will also be investigated. The research sheds light on the question of how personality and subjective validation enable bizarre beliefs and delusions to be maintained even in the light of disconfirmatory evidence.

Subjective validation is also called the 'personal validation effect' because in this process people accept a claim or experience as valid based solely upon personal experiences and/or perception. A person perceives two independent events as having a deeper, hidden relationship because of prior beliefs, expectations, or hypotheses. This subjective validation is a form of 'confirmation bias' whereby supporting data are more heavily weighted than disconfirming data. Subjective validation is a core aspect of people's reports and beliefs concerning the paranormal. For example in experiencing readings by alleged psychics, a person will focus on and/or remember the 'hits' or accurate statements, and forget and/or ignore the 'misses,' or inaccurate statements.

In this way, the person subjectively validates their preconception that there is a 'psychic' or paranormal connection between things in the universe.

Subjective validation may also be used to describe how people can become wedded to, and overconfident about, their prejudices and pet ideas. People, both lay and professional, can easily talk themselves into believing that they are right even when the evidence points towards the possibility that they are wrong. This can lead to problems when defending the idea in the face of challenges by others who are not emotionally wedded to the idea.

Another name for subjective validation is the 'Forer effect,' named after psychologist B. R. Forer who discovered, in 1948, that a person can willingly accept some general or vague description of their personality as being unique to them, even though the same description can be applied equally to everybody. Forer gave a personality test to his students and, without bothering to look at the answers, provided them all with the same general personality analysis extracted from a newspaper astrology column. The analysis read as follows:

> You have a need for other people to like and admire you, and yet you tend to be critical of yourself. While you have some personality weaknesses you are generally able to compensate for them. You have considerable unused capacity that you have not turned to your advantage. Disciplined and self-controlled on the outside, you tend to be worrisome and insecure on the inside. At times you have serious doubts as to whether you have made the right decision or done the right thing. You prefer a certain amount of change and variety and become dissatisfied when hemmed in by restrictions and limitations. You also pride yourself as an independent thinker; and do not accept others' statements without satisfactory proof. But you have found it unwise to be too frank in revealing yourself to others. At times you are extroverted, affable, and sociable, while at other times you are introverted, wary, and reserved. Some of your aspirations tend to be rather unrealistic.

Forer asked his students to rate this analysis and received a highly positive response. Forer's students were convinced that he could 'read' their personalities. This study is easily replicated and the author has done so on numerous occasions. Unfortunately, most Forer-type studies have been conducted only on college students. In the research to be reported here, we used a sample of community volunteers, more representative of the general population.

The Forer effect helps to explain why so many people readily believe that pseudosciences, such as astrology, fortune telling, and graphology, are valid. Marks and Kammann (1980) argued that:

> once a belief or expectation is found, especially one that resolves uncomfortable uncertainty, it biases the observer to notice new information that confirms the belief, and to discount evidence to the contrary. This self-perpetuating mechanism consolidates the original error and builds up an overconfidence in which the arguments of opponents are seen as too fragmentary to undo the adopted belief.

The 'fantasy-prone person', as identified by Wilson and Barber (1983), has frequent involvement with imagination and fantasy, high hypnotic susceptibility, and reports high numbers of paranormal-type experiences (Lynn and Rhue, 1988). Crawley (2002) found significant correlations between the Vividness of Visual Imagery Questionnaire (VVIQ-2; Marks, 1995), the Australian Sheep–Goats Scale (Thalbourne and Delin, 1993), the Revised Paranormal Belief Scale (Tobacyk, 1988), and fantasy proneness, suggesting a common set of characteristics among believers in the paranormal as compared to sceptics. A further relevant construct is that of 'transliminality' defined as a 'hypothesized tendency for psychosocial material to cross (trans) the threshold (limen) into or out of consciousness' (Thalbourne, 2000, p. 31). These concepts, and the theoretical links between them, provide the background for the current research.

Large-scale surveys have revealed that a large proportion of the general population believes in paranormal phenomena. A recent Gallup poll (2001) has found that, overall, over a half or more of Americans believe in the two following issues: psychic or spiritual healing, and extrasensory perception (ESP). In addition, a third or more believe in things such as haunted houses, possession by the devil, ghosts, telepathy, extraterrestrial beings having visited earth, and clairvoyance. The situation is quite similar in the UK and elsewhere in Europe.

Paranormal beliefs are usually defined as experiences which, if true, would involve processes that are, in principle, outside the realm of human capabilities as presently conceived by science. Regardless of whether these phenomena are real or not, they have important theoretical and clinical implications. A number of studies have indicated a link between schizotypy and paranormal belief (Thalbourne *et al.*, 1997; Thalbourne, 1994; Thalbourne and Delin, 1994). One of the first reports was by Windholz and Diamant (1974), who found that believers in the paranormal scored higher on the hypomania and schizophrenia scales of the MMPI. Hence, our first aim was to replicate the finding that people scoring highly on paranormal belief scales will score highly on a schizotypy questionnaire. However, as schizotypy is a multidimensional construct, and the questionnaires which we used measured a number of different aspects of schizotypy, we planned to carry out a more fine-grained analysis of exactly what aspects of schizotypy can predict paranormal belief.

In addition to the above, we planned to take the study a step further by examining the influence of different types of schizotypy in a paranormal context. Claridge (1985) proposed a continuum model of schizophrenia, whereby latent vulnerability to schizophrenia is displayed in the form of a continuum of cognitive and personality traits that can exist without the overt expression of illness. The model proposes a normal distribution of latency to schizophrenia in the general population, ranging from low at one extreme to overt schizophrenia at the other. Schizotypy thus refers to an individual's susceptibility to display schizophrenic symptomatology. One of the core symptoms of schizophrenia is delusions; these are stable, unshakeable ideas, which are held with extraordinary conviction.

Given that we are making the assumption that schizotypy is a dimensional correlate of schizophrenia we would expect individuals high in this construct to behave differently from those scoring low. In particular, as mentioned above, some schizophrenic patients display delusions which are incorrigibly held. Therefore, we expected individuals high in certain aspects of schizotypy to maintain their prior beliefs significantly longer than individuals low in schizotypy when given evidence to the contrary.

Recent research

This project focused upon the psychological characteristics of people who believe or do not believe in psi, independently of the issue of whether or not the phenomena are real.

Hypotheses

Previous research suggested that subjective validation is strongly associated with beliefs in the paranormal even when the evidence is equivocal or contrary to the paranormal claim (Marks, 2000). The first hypothesis (H1) is that beliefs in the paranormal are maintained because of subjective validation. A method of assessing subjective validation, developed in pilot studies, is described below. In addition, we test four hypotheses concerning the influence of personality characteristics on paranormal beliefs. The hypotheses are summarized below.

People who form and maintain paranormal beliefs are hypothesized to be high scorers in tests or scales assessing:

H1 subjective validation

H2 schizotypy

H3 fantasizing

H4 vividness of imagery

Furthermore we hypothesized that:

H5 the above characteristics will be positively correlated.

Method

Pilot study

The methods were piloted in a study carried out at Cardiff University with 24 participants in collaboration with Professor Robert J. Snowden, Dr Nicola Gray, and Lisa H. Evans. The pilot study formed the basis for the larger-scale study. Improvements to the procedures were made following the pilot study.

Sample

There were 120 participants who were interested in the paranormal and/or believed that they were psychic. All participants were above 18 years of age with a range 18–59 and a mean age of 24 years. Sixty-two per cent were females and 38 per cent were males. There were two experimenters, both of whom were trained by the principal investigator.

Materials

To assess paranormal beliefs, two questionnaires were administered. The first one was the Australian Sheep–Goat Scale (Thalbourne and Delin, 1993) and the second was the Revised Paranormal Belief Scale (R-PBS; Tobacyk, 1988). In the Australian Sheep–Goat Scale participants were asked to indicate the extent to which they agreed or disagreed with statements by circling a true/false response. The R-PBS was measured on a 7-point scale, ranging from strongly disagree to strongly agree. This questionnaire consisted of six sub-scales: (1) traditional religious belief, (2) psi, (3) witchcraft, (4) superstition, (5) spiritualism, (6) extraordinary life events, and (7) precognition. The experimenters also completed the Australian Sheep–Goat Scale and the Revised Paranormal Belief Scale.

To assess schizotypy, the Oxford–Liverpool Inventory of Feelings and Experiences (O-LIFE; Mason *et al.*, 1995) was utilized. This assessment tool measures four dimensions of schizotypy (introvertive anhedonia, unusual experiences, impulsive non-conformity, and cognitive disorganization). Introvertive anhedonia describes a lack of enjoyment from social activities and suggests a dislike of emotional and physical intimacy. Unusual experiences contain items on hallucinatory and magical thinking. Impulsive non-conformity describes self-abusive and reckless behaviours. Lastly, cognitive disorganization refers to difficulties with attention and concentration.

To assess fantasizing we used the Wilson–Barber Inventory of Childhood Memories and Imaginings: Children's Form (Myers, 1983). To assess imagery vividness, we used the Vividness of Visual Imagery Questionnaire (VVIQ;

Marks, 1973). Finally, to assess transliminality, we used the Transliminality Scale, Form B (Thalbourne, 1998). These last three questionnaires were used as indicators of participants' imaging and fantasizing styles.

Procedure

The procedure was in four phases: (1) obtaining of informed consent; (2) completion of questionnaires; (3) completion of the card-guessing task; and (4) de-briefing.

Phase (1): participants were first given an information sheet and a consent form to complete.

Phase (2): they completed the above questionnaires in counterbalanced order.

Phase (3): participants carried out the card-guessing phase of the experiment. During the card guessing phase of the experiment a pack of 40 especially organized Zener Cards was used. These cards had five different designs on them: cross, star, circle, square, and three wavy lines. Sitting on opposite sides of a table an experimenter and the participant interacted as cards were pulled from the pack by the experimenter. The cards were swiftly pulled from the top or the back of the pack using a prearranged, non-randomized pack. The participant was allowed to cut the pack but not in a way that disturbed the prearranged sequence. On each of 40 trials the participant had to predict which card was coming next, out of a possible five. After each guess they stated how confident they were on a scale of 1–100 (1 being not confident at all and 100 being totally confident). Participants were asked to give confidence ratings for each of the 40 trials.

As noted above, the sequence of cards was manipulated artificially to provide false feedback. The feedback indicated that their predictions were above chance level in the first block of 20 trials. If the normal rules of probability applied, then it would be expected that participants could obtain approximately four correct predictions out of 20 (an average of 1 in 5 or 20 per cent). However, in the first block of 20 trials a sleight-of-hand was performed, which tended to increase the participants' prediction rate to eight out of 20 or 40 per cent. After this, participants were given a second 20-trial block, in which the cards were manipulated to decrease the prediction rate.

Participants were asked to fill out a brief questionnaire to assess what they thought was happening during the study and to assess their beliefs in the their psychic abilities at the end of the study. They were asked two questions: (a) Are you psychic? (b) What kind of forces do you think you have when you do this kind of task? Each question could receive a score ranging from 0 to 2. Participants receiving 0 did not believe that they were psychic, those receiving a 1 did not know whether they had any psychic abilities, and, lastly, participants scoring 2 believed themselves to be psychic. Total scores for these two items ranged from 0 to 4. Participants scoring above 2 were classified as self-proclaimed psychic believers.

Finally, participants were given a fair test using a pack of 25 Zener cards. Feedback was given accurately and the participant was informed at the end how many correct guesses they had achieved.

Phase (4): participants were debriefed. The methods used were explained and the participants received the opportunity to ask any questions about what had taken place. Participants getting high prediction scores – having being informed of the deception – might have felt a little disappointment but there was no evidence that anybody suffered a significant amount of stress. Those participants who did not believe that they were psychic in the first place had this belief confirmed, whereas participants who believed that they were psychic continued to believe this. Most of the participants who had faith in their psychic abilities and scored low on the Zener cards thought that the only important factor affecting their performance was the laboratory conditions, not that they had been manipulated. Participants were given a telephone number to call if they had any further questions or issues to raise. In discussing the experiment with the participants, no untoward negative impacts were evident. Indeed the participants were in general amused and/or bemused by their results, but, as we shall see below, very few changed their beliefs as a result of the investigation.

Results

Subjective validation: the average correct prediction rates for the three trial blocks are given in Table 2.1. As the participants' overall confidence remained high in spite of the markedly reduced performance in the second and third blocks of trials, this indicates a strong subjective validation effect. The range in confidence scores was relatively high and we used the average confidence on block 2 as a measure of subjective validation (SV).

Paranormal beliefs: means and standard deviations of scores on the Australian S-G and R-PBS are presented in Table 2.2. The mean and standard deviations (SD) for the present population are compared to the norms on the R-PBS for university students in the southern United States. The present population scored higher in the R-PBS than did university students in the southern United States.

Table 2.1 Average correct prediction rates

Trial block	Correct guesses		Confidence	
	Mean (MCE)	SD	Mean	SD
1 (20 cards)	7.70 (4.00)	1.24	32.3	4.8
2 (20 cards)	1.57 (4.00)	1.12	31.8	5.1
3 (40 cards)	8.10 (8.00)	1.43	32.3	5.8

MCE = mean chance expectation

Table 2.2 Means and standard deviations for the Revised Paranormal Belief Scale (R-PBS) and the Australian Sheep–Goats (S-G) scale

	Mean	SD
Australian S-G	11.67	3.97
R-PBS present sample	103.45	21.10
R-PBS university students US	89.10	21.90

Table 2.3 Means and standard deviations for the O-LIFE scale

Scale	Mason *et al.* (1995)		Current sample	
	Mean	SD	Mean	SD
Unusual experiences	9.7	6.7	12.8	7.08
Cognitive disorganization	11.6	5.8	10.12	5.75
Introvertive anhedonia	6.1	4.6	6.35	4.76
Impulsive non-conformity	9.1	4.3	6.24	4.30

Schizotypy: the means and SD for the O-LIFE questionnaire are reported in Table 2.3. The mean and SD reported for the present population are compared with the norms used in the Mason, Claridge, and Jackson (1995) study. Mason *et al.* (1995) obtained similar scores to the present sample, although the latter did score higher in the unusual experiences dimension of the O-LIFE.

Imagery and fantasy: scores showed wide variability but were well within the range observed in other similar samples (Table 2.4).

Test of hypotheses

H1: predicted relationship between psychic beliefs and subjective valida-tion. Self-proclaimed psychic beliefs were assessed by scoring the questions in

Table 2.4 Means and standard deviations on the Vividness of Visual Imagery Questionnaire (VVIQ) and Wilson–Barber Inventory (WBI)

Questionnaire	Mean	SD
VVIQ-2	80.58	12.45
WBICMI-CF	16.78	6.39

Table 2.5 Correlations between schizotypy scales and psychic beliefs

Schizotypy scale	r	p
Unusual	0.432	<0.001
Cognitive disorganization	0.301	<0.001
Introvertive anhedonia	−0.449	<0.001
Impulsive non-conformity	0.16	NS

phase (3) of the procedure: (a) Are you psychic? (b) What kind of forces do you think you have when you do this kind of task? The correlation between SV and psychic beliefs was 0.64 (df = 118; p < 0.001). This finding shows that persons with high scores in subjective validation also had a strong tendency to proclaim psychic powers.

H2: predicted relationship between psychic beliefs and schizotypy scales. A significant association occurred between the participants' scores on three of the schizotype scales and beliefs in their psychic abilities (Table 2.5).

H3: predicted relationship between psychic beliefs and fantasizing. The correlation between the Wilson–Barber Inventory and psychic beliefs was 0.46 (p < 0.001), confirming the hypothesis.

H4: predicted relationship between psychic beliefs and vividness of imagery. The correlation between the VVIQ-2 and psychic beliefs was 0.58, confirming the hypothesis.

H5: predicted relationship between the characteristics of subjective validation, schizotypy, fantasizing, and vividness of imagery. The correlation matrix for the eight variables is given in Table 2.6 below. It can be seen that the majority of correlations are positive, providing confirmation of the hypothesis.

Discussion

All five of the study hypotheses were confirmed by the experimental data. This study has helped to identify the characteristics of people who strongly believe

Table 2.6 Correlations between psychic belief, subjective validation, schizotypy fantasizing and imagery

	Psychic beliefs	Subjective validation	Introvertive anhedonia	Unusual experiences	Impulsive non-conformity	Cognitive disorganization	WBI	VVIQ-2
Psychic beliefs	—	0.642	0.178	0.434	0.410	0.378	0.463	0.579
Subjective validation		—	−0.389	0.448	0.009	0.336	0.238	0.390
Introvertive anhedonia			—	−0.190	0.107	0.198	0.008	−0.105
Unusual experiences				—	−0.437	0.612	0.594	0.634
Impulsive non-conformity					—	0.421	0.005	0.386
Cognitive disorganization						—	0.361	0.499
WBI							—	0.683

WBI = Wilson–Barber Inventory; VVIQ = Vividness of Visual Imagery Questionnaire in personal psychic powers in spite of disconfirmation of their beliefs by actual physical events. Psychic believers have a strong tendency to subjectively validate and have personality characteristics that are linked to schizotypy. In accordance with a number of studies, which have indicated a link between schizotypy and paranormal belief (Thalbourne *et al.*, 1997; Thalbourne, 1994; Thalbourne and Delin, 1994), the present investigation obtained an association between paranormal beliefs and specific dimensions of schizotypy personalities.

Previous research has indicated that beliefs in the paranormal are a consequence of confirmation biases and wishful thinking which have no basis in objective facts and independent observation (Marks and Kammann, 1980; Marks, 1986; Marks, 2000). The present study suggests that those who continue to believe in psychic powers, even when their beliefs are discredited by evidence, have personality characteristics that are continuous with those observed in schizophrenics, fantasizers, and people with vivid imagery. This is a result which will not surprise many scientists and sceptics of the paranormal. However, it is a result that should give pause to those who continue to claim the existence of powers and phenomena for which there is no objective evidence.

Acknowledgements

I thank Dr Luis Portela and the Fundação Bial for generous support. I would like to acknowledge the collaboration of Professor Robert J. Snowden, Dr Nicola Gray and Lisa H. Evans of Cardiff University in the formative stages of this research. Anastasia Soureti and Yoriko Taniguchi provided assistance in data collection. I dedicate this research to the memory of the late Robert Morris, a leading researcher of the paranormal.

References

Claridge, G (1985). *Origins of mental health*. Oxford: Blackwell.

Crawley, SE (2002). *Daydream believers?* PhD thesis, Goldsmiths College, London University.

Lynn and Rhue (1988). Fantasy proneness, hypnosis, developmental antecedents and psychopathology. *American Psychologist*, **43**, 35–44.

Marks, D (2000). *The psychology of the psychic*, 2nd edn. Amherst: Prometheus Books.

Marks, D and Kammann, R (1980). *The psychology of the psychic*. Buffalo: Prometheus Books.

Marks, DF (1973). Visual imagery differences in the recall of pictures. *British Journal of Psychology*, **64**, 17–24.

Marks, DF (1986). Investigating the paranormal. *Nature*, **320**, 119–124.

Marks, DF (1995). New directions for mental imagery research. *Journal of Mental Imagery*, **19**, 153–167.

Mason, O, Claridge, C and Jackson, M (1995). New scales for the assessment of schizotypy. *Personality and Individual Differences*, **18**, 7–13.

Myers, SA (1983). The Wilson-Barber inventory of childhood memories and imaginings: Children's form and norms for 1337 children and adolescents. *Journal of Mental Imagery*, **7**, 196–205.

Thalbourne, MA (1994). Belief in the paranormal and its relationship to schizophrenia-relevant measures: a confirmatory study. *British Journal of Clinical Psychology*, **33**, 78–80.

Thalbourne, MA (2000). Transliminality: A review. *International Journal of Parapsychology*, **11**, 1–34.

Thalbourne, MA, Bartemucci, L, Delin, PS, Fox, B and Nofi, O (1997). Transliminality: its nature and correlates. *Journal of the American Society for Physical Research*, **91**, 305–331.

Thalbourne, MA and Delin, PS (1994). A common thread underlying belief in the paranormal, creative personality, mystical experience and psychopathology. *Journal of Parapsychology*, **58**, 3–38.

Tobacyk, JJ (1988). *A revised paranormal belief scale*. Unpublished manuscript, Louisiana Tech University, Ruston, LA.

Wilson, S and Barber, TX (1983). The Fantasy prone personality. In AA Sheikh (ed.) *Imagery Current Theory, Research & Application*. New York: Wiley, pp 340–390.

Windholz, G and Diamant, L (1974). Some personality traits of true believers in extrasensory phenomena. *Bulletin of the Psychonomic Society*, **3**, 125–6.

Chapter 3

The cognitive anthropology of belief

Quinton Deeley

Introduction

Of all disciplines, anthropology has most concerned itself with understanding two sources of constraint on cognition and behaviour: those due to membership of the humans species, and those due to membership of particular societies or social groups. For much of the twentieth century, species constraints were the focus of physical or biological anthropology, while cultural constraints were the focus of social anthropology (Durham, 1991). In recent years, the picture has become more complex, partly due to the advent of new disciplines (for example sociobiology and evolutionary psychology), and partly because of greater interdisciplinary exchanges. In this chapter I will discuss various developments that have come to be termed 'cognitive anthropology', focusing on the accounts they give of the 'power of belief', particularly in relation to beliefs about illness and its treatment. To begin, we will consider a fundamental aspect of beliefs confronting any cross-cultural observer: their extreme diversity.

Medical pluralism and the diversity of beliefs

It is common in all human cultures (including those of the West) for different conceptions of illness and modes of treatment to be pursued simultaneously or at different times in relation to illness. Anthropologists use the term *medical pluralism* to describe this phenomenon (Good, 1995; Kleinman, 1988a, b). In India, for example, a range of models of illness and its treatment are often drawn on serially or in parallel by sick individuals and their close community (Deeley, 1999; 2000). In addition to 'allopathic' (biomedical) approaches, other explanations and/or modes of treatment include: the indigenous humoral medicine of Ayurveda; attribution of illness to spirit possession and the enlistment of a *brahmin* priest to perform a healing ceremony or exorcism (*puja*); consultation of possession oracles; homeopathy;

illness as punishment for failure to fulfil a religious vow or duty; and consultation with astrologers (Leslie and Young, 1992). If the list seems extensive, consider that in the UK most of the above are not merely present within communities with links to the Indian subcontinent, but some of them (e.g. Ayurveda, homeopathy) increasingly inform understandings of, and responses to, illness in the wider society. Diverse illness models and treatments have not merely been introduced by migrant communities but are also actively sought out and developed by other groups in society, including the majority white British population. Indeed, the range of approaches in the UK which make some claim to be able to explain, prevent, treat (or cause) various kinds of illness and misfortune is probably impossible to list exhaustively, although examples might include: evangelical Christianity, acupuncture, aromatherapy, macrobiotic diets, Trancendental Mediation (TM), scientology, and voodoo (noting that to list them as such is not to imply equivalence between them, but to illustrate their diversity) (Littlewood, 2002; Littlewood and Lipsedge, 1989).

This fact of medical pluralism raises fundamental questions: how do human beings acquire such diverse beliefs about illness and its treatment? And, more broadly, in what ways do species-level constraints interact with cultural and individual constraints on the formation of beliefs? For the purposes of this chapter, we will use Sperber's definition, in which belief is 'a disposition to express, assent to, or otherwise act in accordance with some proposition' (Sperber, 1996, p. 86). Note that this definition encompasses consciously held beliefs as well as presuppositions that might influence cognition below the level of awareness.

Extrapersonal and intrapersonal constraints on cognition and behaviour

A distinction between 'extrapersonal' and 'intrapersonal' constraints on cognition is fundamental to understanding long-standing debates about the relations between culture and cognition, and hence of the relations between culture and belief. Hannerz described the distinction in the following terms:

> . . . culture has two kinds of loci, and the cultural process takes place in their ongoing inter-relations. On the one hand, culture resides in a set of public meaningful forms, which can most often be seen or heard, or are somewhat less frequently known through touch, smell, or taste, if not through some combination of senses. On the other hand, these overt forms are only rendered meaningful because human minds contain the instruments for their interpretation. The cultural flow thus consists of the externalizations of meaning which individuals produce through arrangements of overt forms, and the interpretations which individuals made of such displays – those of others as well as their own

(quoted in Strauss and Quinn, 1997, p. 10).

Theoretical approaches in social and cultural anthropology in the twentieth century tended to assert the priority of culture (the extrapersonal realm) in constraining individual behaviour (Durham, 1991). As the British social anthropologist Victor Turner put it, 'social anthropologists of my generation were taught that all human behaviour is the result of social conditioning' (Turner, 1983). Along with this *cultural determinism*, 'cultures' themselves tended to be conceived as strongly individuated (by analogy with different languages), bounded, relatively static, coherent systems of meaning, social roles, relations, artefacts, institutions (depending on theoretical emphasis – see, for example, Ortner, 1984). Strong claims for *cultural relativism* entailed that the scope for intercultural variation was almost indefinite, with few constraints on cognition imposed by intrapersonal factors (for example genes, learning biases, or species-typical cognitive mechanisms) (Hollis and Lukes, 1982). Individual differences tended to be attributed to extrapersonal factors such as differences in social role expectations. Hence, understanding an individual's 'beliefs' (world-view) involved understanding the culture to which they belonged, which could be described using the convention of the 'ethnographic present' – for example, 'the X believe that illness is caused by spirits'.

Anthropologists have subjected strong versions of such 'culturalism' to a number of criticisms, whilst attempting to preserve the insights gained from the discipline's attention to describing and modelling the extrapersonal realm. As Strauss and Quinn put it,

> we have learned how problematic it is, in a world of shifting and multiple identities, to label any set of people as 'the X'. But to a greater extent the problem lies with the phrase 'the culture of the X'. In our discipline's past, such descriptions have too often made it sound as if all the X thought, felt, and acted the same way, had shared this way of life for centuries and would have continued in their traditional ways, unchanged, if colonial education and modern mass media had not intervened. Past descriptions, too, sometimes missed the extent to which the story they told about traditional cultural values and practices was the interested account of one powerful class or faction or a public 'for show' version that hid alternative accounts, challenges to the powerful, or even mundane, widely held practices and understandings that contradicted informants' conscious beliefs about what they were doing
>
> (Strauss and Quinn, 1997, p. 3).

The cognitive anthropology of 'belief'

In the wake of such criticisms, some anthropologists have reconceptualized 'culture', and used models derived from cognitive and evolutionary psychology to specify the 'intrapersonal' processes involved in the acquisition of beliefs.

The cognitive anthropologist Sperber distinguishes two kinds of representation. *Mental* (or *internal*) representations exist in the minds and brains of individuals – examples include beliefs, memories, and intentions. *Public* (or *external*) representations exist in the environment: 'signals, utterances, texts and pictures are all public representations' (Sperber, 1996, p. 24). They acquire or convey meaning when they are interpreted in terms of mental representations.

On this basis, Sperber has proposed an 'epidemiological' approach to culture, in which:

> cultural facts are . . . distributions of causally linked mental and public facts in a human population. More specifically, chains of interaction – of communication in particular – may distribute similar mental representations and similar public productions (such as behaviors and artifacts) throughout a population. Types of mental representations and public productions that are stabilized through such causal chains, are in fact, what we recognize as cultural
>
> (Sperber and Hirschfeld, 2001, p. cxxii).

This 'epidemiological' view may seem similar to Dawkin's atomistic theory of 'memes' (items of cultural information constituting a 'meme pool', by analogy with genes in a gene pool) (Dawkins, 1976). Yet Sperber criticizes the meme theory's account of cultural transmission, which extends the analogy with genetics to imply a 'decoding' and 'copying' model of items of cultural information from mind to mind. By contrast, Sperber's version of cognitive anthropology views human communication as based on inferential interpretation of communicative acts rather than the decoding and replication of representations (Sperber and Hirschfeld, 2001).

On this basis, Sperber distinguishes two kinds of 'belief'. *Intuitive beliefs* are 'intuitive in the sense that they are typically the product of spontaneous and unconscious perceptual and inferential processes' (Sperber, 1996, p. 89). Intuitive beliefs are viewed as generated by the rapid, automatic assumptions and inferential processes of evolved mental modules (Sperber, 1996). Humans reason about objects in ways that are distinct for the category of things to which an object belongs; these distinctive forms of reasoning are termed 'naïve theories' (Sperber, 1996). For example 'the spontaneous expectations of not only infants but also adults about the unity, boundaries, and persistence of physical objects may be based on a rather rigid naïve physics' (Sperber and Hirschfeld, 2001). Other domains with their own conceptual mechanisms include theory of mind/naïve psychology (which interprets agentive behaviour in terms of a 'belief-desire psychology'), and folk biology (which partitions and explains living things in terms of biological principles like growth, inheritance, and bodily function) (Sperber and Hirschfeld, 2001).

Reflective beliefs, by contrast, are based on interpretation, the capacity of human minds to re-represent or reflect on concepts. He argues that they do not form a well-defined category, but rather 'come embedded in intuitive beliefs (or since there can be multiple embeddings, in other reflective beliefs). They cause belief behaviours because, one way or another, the belief in which they are embedded validates them' (Sperber, 1996, p. 89).

Explaining belief in the supernatural

Boyer has applied this approach to explaining religious beliefs, which would include the use of supernatural concepts and related practices to explain and treat illness. The approach can be illustrated by applying it to a case study described by Deeley (1999), the main points of which are summarized below, based on an illness narrative elicited from the brother of an inpatient at the All India Institute of Medical Sciences in New Delhi. He recounted his perspective on the causes and course of illness of his younger sister, who was an inpatient on the psychiatry ward, diagnosed with hysterical aphonia and paralysis. His sister had fallen ill with fever after retaking an English proficiency exam. She attended the local hospital, and various investigations including a lumbar puncture were performed. No cause of her fever was found, and she was discharged home. Shortly afterwards, she became bed-bound, unable to walk or talk, and had to be fed, dressed, and helped to the toilet. The family believed that the lumbar puncture may have caused her problems. After several weeks the family arranged a *puja* (healing ceremony) with a local *Brahmin* priest. During the ceremony, she gesticulated for a pen and paper. She began to write in what appeared to be Urdu, which her Hindi speaking family could not read (and which she herself did not know). They asked her to write in Hindi. She wrote that that she had been taken over by the spirit of a Muslim man (hence Urdu) who (she wrote) had been strangled to death in the village the previous year. This was why she was unable to speak. She stood and prayed like a Muslim man for one hour. The priest said she would be better in one month. The family accepted her attribution of her problems to spirit possession. In the following weeks she regained abilities such as feeding herself, but remained mute. Then her functioning deteriorated, and her family no longer believed she had been possessed because of her failure to recover. She was referred to a national centre, AIIMS in New Delhi, where neurologists diagnosed hysterical aphonia and paralysis, and referred her for inpatient treatment on the psychiatry ward. At the time of interview the brother said that because the treatment with the doctor was ineffective, the family were 'forced to believe in the spirit. He added that now they believed the doctors, though he also repeated that his family believed her problems were caused by the lumbar puncture received at the time of the fever' (Deeley, 1999, p. 113, see original for full version).

What makes the notion of spirit possession sufficiently credible for it to be invoked by the young woman in the context of a healing ceremony, and for family members to accept it (believe it), even if only provisionally?

In Boyer's account of religious belief, supernatural concepts acquire salience by selectively violating domain-based assumptions about the category of things to which they ostensibly belong. Like Sperber, Boyer proposes distinct conceptual domains and inference-mechanisms that interpret the broad categories of objects to be found in the world (PERSONS, ARTEFACTS, ANIMALS, PLANTS). Each category is associated with an 'intuitive ontology', a naïve theory about the properties of the things it contains (exemplified above with reference to Sperber's 'naïve theories').

Given this cognitive background, 'religious concepts are constrained by intuitive ontologies in two different ways: (1) they include explicit *violations* of intuitive expectations, and (2) they tacitly activate a *background* of non-violated default expectations' (Boyer, 2000, p. 101, Boyer, 2002, 2003; Barrett, 2000).

He then proposes the following 'template' for supernatural concepts:

[0] a lexical label

[1] a pointer to a particular ontological category

[2] an explicit representation of a violation of intuitive expectations, either:

    [2a] a *breach* of relevant expectations for the category, or

    [2b] a *transfer* of expectations associated with another category

[3] a link to (non-violated) default expectations for the category

[4] a slot for additional encyclopaedic information (Boyer, 2000, p. 101).

We can apply this to the notion of spirit possession in the narrative described above as follows:

[0] 'spirit' (the English word was chosen by the translators from Hindi)

[1] PERSON

[2] an explicit representation of a violation of intuitive expectations, in this case:

    [2a] it survives death and does not need a body to exist; it can possess the living and cause disabilities or other problems

[3] it exhibits a 'belief-desire' psychology of seeking vengeance, an intelligible motive given that:

[4] it is the spirit of a Muslim man strangled in the village the previous year.

A key implication of this approach is that violation of intuitive expectations for a category is limited: 'a supernatural being with too few unexpected qualities is not attention demanding and thus not memorable. One with too many unexpected qualities is too information rich to be memorable' (Sperber and Hirschfeld, 2001, p. cxxi). Research on memory for concepts has shown that concepts with a counterintuitive feature (e.g. a dog that passes through solid objects) are more memorable than either fully intuitive concepts (e.g. a brown dog) or bizarre concepts that violate basic, rather than category level, assumptions (e.g. a dog that weighs five tons) (see Barrett, 2000; Boyer, 2000, and for further evidence cited to support the existence of species-typical, early-developed, domain-specific structures of intuitive ontology that underpin religious conceptual templates and memory organization).

'Conceptual salience' and 'belief'

While concepts that minimally violate intuitive expectations may be salient and memorable, this does not necessarily make them *believable*. The characters and events of Greek mythology produce interesting and memorable stories, but few if any now *believe* that the Cyclops really exists. So what, in this view, motivates *belief*, in Sperber's sense of 'a disposition to express, assent to, or otherwise act in accordance with some proposition' (Sperber, 1996, p. 86)?

In *Religion Explained* (Boyer, 2002), Boyer attributes the credibility of supernatural concepts to two kinds of cognitive phenomena – the *aggregate relevance* of concepts, interacting with a suite of minor 'reasoning errors', departures from strict rationality that increase the apparent plausibility of supernatural concepts.

The 'aggregate relevance' of a supernatural belief refers to the way in which a variety of cognitive processes and mechanisms contribute to its plausibility, with no one mechanism likely to be sufficient in its own right. On this view, religious ideas meet the 'entry requirements' for many different kinds of domain-based reasoning, and gain plausibility because of the diverse inferences that they allow. Since gods, ancestors, and spirits belong to the ontological category of PERSONS, they automatically qualify for all of the kinds of reasoning routinely applied to PERSONS in ordinary cognition, with some changes in keeping with the features that violate domain assumptions. Hence, the intuitive-psychology system treats ancestors (or spirits or gods) as intentional agents, the exchange system treats them as exchange partners, the moral system treats them as potential witnesses to moral actions, the Person File system treats them as distinct individuals (paraphrasing Boyer, 2002, p. 361). As Boyer continues, 'this means that quite a lot of mental work is going on, producing specific inferences about the ancestors [or spirits or gods] without ever requiring explicit general statements to the effect that, for example, "there really are invisible ancestors around", "they are dead people", "they have powers" etc.' (brackets inserted; Boyer, 2002, p. 361). Boyer argues that the inferential relevance of supernatural agents is vastly increased by regarding them as 'perfect access' intentional agents – in other words, knowing what is truly the case – since they can be presumed to take an interest in a far wider range of events than real people could possibly know about (Boyer, 2002, p. 362). This inferential relevance, coupled with a universal cognitive tendency to overascribe intentional agency when interpreting events (Guthrie, 1980), explains why the counterintuitive concepts of supernatural beings are more common than non-intentional counterintuitive objects, such as invisible sofas. The latter have much less inferential relevance (Boyer, 2002; Barrett, 2000).

In addition to this 'aggregate relevance', supernatural concepts are accepted because of the commission of common reasoning errors – the list cited by Boyer includes *consensus effects* within the social group; *false consensus effects* (wrongly judging one's own idiosyncratic conception of supernatural concepts to be shared by others); *generation effects* (enhanced memory for self-generated understandings of supernatural concepts); *source monitoring defects* (misattribution to oneself of claims about experiences which apparently confirm the existence and activities of supernatural agents); *confirmation bias* (recollection of instances of apparent confirmation of a supernatural belief, but not of disconfirmations); *cognitive dissonance reduction* (adjustment of expectations in the light of experience which contradicts initial expectations, in order to preserve a belief) (paraphrasing Boyer, 2002, p. 346 f.).

Critique of the model

Boyer's model entails that the various inference systems constitute a 'standard architecture that we all have by being members of the species' (Boyer, 2000, p. 154). In this view, group level processes provide the superficial, local conceptual content for inference systems, while the species-typical inference systems that process this local content have a rigid, encapsulated design. Their constituent processes can be discovered by cognitive research, but are not accessible to conscious introspection. By analogy with generative grammar, the surface structures of religious belief are local, while the deep structures (the templates and inference systems) are universal. Flexibility in processing is introduced by the selective activation and deactivation of inference systems in accordance with the properties of information presented for processing. Ontological categories function as 'switches' that route conceptual processing through the relevant inference systems (Boyer, 2002, p. 128). Thus, the example cited above of how notions of gods, spirits, and ancestors are processed entails that by ostensibly belonging to the ontological category of PERSONS, specific subsets of all of the potentially available inference systems (the social exchange system, the person file system, etc.) are activated as necessary to generate relevant inferences. Nevertheless, the inference systems themselves remain encapsulated, unconscious, and shared by all normal members of the species.

Questions confronting Boyer's model will be considered here, in order to indicate alternative ways of understanding the social embeddedness of cognition, including belief. Note that these criticisms are relevant to those versions of evolutionary psychology and cognitive psychology that share the same assumptions about cognition outlined above.

As an initial point, the reasoning errors cited by Boyer as influencing religious belief formation are present in relation to belief in other kinds of concepts and propositions, including those of medicine. All of the reasoning errors could conceivably contribute to the belief of a doctor who was part of a group that advocated, say, megavitamin treatment for flu on the basis of a theory and some anecdotal experience. Indeed, the procedures of evidence-based medicine are designed to limit the effects of such errors and biases. Hence, reasoning errors cannot *differentially* explain beliefs in supernatural concepts as opposed to any other kind of concept even if they contribute in some circumstances.

Relations between concepts and inference systems

More fundamentally, Boyer's model raises the question of what kinds of conceptual systems there are, and how they relate to each other. Inference systems relating to some domains, and the competences they support, do not operate uniformly within all members of the species. For example reading and complex mathematics depend on teaching methods that were invented in specific cultural settings, and were certainly not present in our environment of evolutionary adaptedness. Their respective skills and concepts become internalized through education. Hence, at least for some domains and abilities, group differences do make a difference to the 'deep' structures (conceptual templates and inference systems) as well as the 'surface' structures (conceptual content) of cognition.

Boyer accepts this, but argues that the key inference systems tapped by religious concepts are more universal than those supporting abilities such as local versions of reading and mathematics, and develop without requiring formal instruction or education (Boyer, 2002, p. 211). Even if we accept this, the existence of group-specific as well as species-typical concepts and inference systems raises the question of how they are functionally integrated during development and on-line cognition. If Boyer's model demonstrated that universal systems consistently operated independently of group level differences, we might accept that the account of religious concepts is valid. Alternatively, if reasoning about and interpretation of events showed the effects of inferential and associative linkages between locally acquired supernatural concepts and other concepts, then we might conclude that Boyer's model should be substantially qualified. We would have to accept that group differences do make a difference to religious cognition, not just at the 'surface' level of conceptual content, but at the 'deep' level of conceptual structure, inferential relations, motivation, and belief. So an important question is: are there grounds for believing that reasoning about supernatural beings, and belief in supernatural beings, is influenced by locally acquired, superordinate inferential structures that organize the relations between concepts?

Consider, for example, a cross-cultural study that demonstrated that counter-intuitive concepts do indeed seem to be more memorable than control tasks in different populations (Boyer and Ramble, 2001). The study used concepts that were not present in religions familiar to the subjects, but also showed that cultural familiarity with some types of domain-level violations made other types more salient (Boyer and Ramble, 2001). This suggests a local knowledge effect on memory formation, whereby familiarity with a structural type (rather than a specific concept) *decreases* salience. More importantly, though, the study was of memory for unfamiliar concepts, rather than locally familiar concepts that had acquired extensive associative linkages with other concepts and beliefs. It was not, therefore, a study of enculturated beliefs, but rather a study of memory for concepts that had not been incorporated into local knowledge structures. The point here relates to the cognitive difference between concepts that share a structural similarity with religious concepts, and religious concepts that have been internalized through cultural learning. Studies of the former cannot be taken as studies of the latter, if we consider that enculturation itself modifies features of conceptual processing such as motivational salience, inferential relations, and plausibility.

Studies that have been conducted on cognition about divine beings that *are* objects of belief for experimental participants have shown a discrepancy between complex theological views of the properties of the divine beings, and the simpler and more anthropomorphic inferences made about the same divine beings during problem solving and causal reasoning tasks (Barrett and Keil, 1996; Barrett, 2000). This is taken as support for the idea that explicitly held theological ideas about God or gods are distorted and simplified to conform to the expectations of intuitive ontologies (Barrett, 2000). Again, though, an adequate model of such constrained religious reasoning must also be able to account for how its outputs (e.g. a specific causal attribution that an illness is due, say, to punishment by God for failure to fulfil a vow) – relate to inferences made on the basis of other conceptual schemata (e.g. that it is due to lumbar puncture, infection, or even 'hysteria'). The questions of how the outputs of such encapsulated processes relate both to explicit reasoning and judgements about the plausibility and motivational salience of specific ideas remain to be answered.

Explaining group differences in beliefs

A related question concerns how cognition about the supernatural is constrained into locally distinctive forms. A species level of explanation may identify constraints on the wide distribution of certain generic kinds of supernatural concepts (gods, ancestors, spirits, for example), but cannot account for how local versions or subsets of such concepts are accepted or rejected. Hence, spirit possession is widely acknowledged as a possible cause of illness in India, but not amongst English Anglicans at the present time, while atheists in India or England are also likely to reject the possibility entirely (see Macdonald (1990) for a period of English history when possession phenomena were more widely accepted). If Boyer's model of universal inference systems as the overriding constraints on religious belief were correct, then one would expect a similar distribution of similar concepts in all populations. Yet this is not the case, as the spirit possession example illustrates. Hence, Boyer's model fails to account for the processes contributing to differences in beliefs between populations, and processes of historical change in beliefs within populations. A theory of these between-group and within-group variations in beliefs would need to account for how the decision rules governing interpretations of events are formed within social groups – for example the locally distinctive way in which the family's interpretation of the young woman's predicament changed. Even if Boyer's model of universal constraints on supernatural concepts is broadly correct, the question of how these mechanisms are incorporated into local knowledge structures, reasoning, and epistemic judgements remains.

Reflective beliefs and intuitive judgements

Accounting for how the plausibility of concepts is determined is a question for all kinds of belief, supernatural or non-supernatural. In the case of non-supernatural conceptions of illness (for example humoral explanations versus biomedical explanations), practitioners in either form of medicine routinely make rapid judgements about the kind of explanation of illness that are ontologically plausible and epistemologically valid. Hence, most contemporary psychiatrists instantly *know* (or believe they know) that a claim that depression is caused by an excess of black bile is implausible, whereas a claim that depression is caused by deficient serotonin neurotransmission *is* plausible. These kinds of rapid judgements about ontology (what exists) and epistemology (what we know, or can know) are made possible by the extensive internalization of related concepts within specific cultural settings (such as medical schools). Similarly, religions transmit (or fail to transmit) local versions of supernatural concepts, amongst other concepts, values, and behaviours (Bowker, 1987). By considering the effects of cultural systems such as medical schools and religions on cognition, we are reinstating extrapersonal constraints on cognition as a focus of inquiry. Further, non-naïve theories such as those of humoral and biomedicine suggest that Boyer may be overstating the functional distinction between intuitive and reflective beliefs, in so far as what may begin in development as reflective beliefs can function as 'intuitive' beliefs (that is, constrain interpretations of novel events and communication in a rapid, unexamined way). Hence, an account is needed of what allows internalized reflective beliefs to constrain judgements about reality in ways that can (for example) override rival supernatural interpretations that enjoy the benefits of salience and aggregate relevance. Note that the inferential relations between these non-intuitive theories (humoral theories, biomedical theories) and counterintuitive theories (spirit possession) are established within social groups, and certainly cannot be predicted from species membership alone.

Analytic and analogical modes of thought

There are significant culturally acquired inferential links between items belonging to the same and/or different ontological categories. For example astrology posits causal influence between the movements of stars and planets and human affairs, including the psychological, social, and political realms (choosing an auspicious date for a wedding or nuclear arms negotiations), and the physical realm of unsolicited illness or injury (explaining injury due to an accident). Again, these inferential links cannot be predicted from category membership alone, but require attention to local understandings of the world. Indeed, in many societies the formation of analogical or correlative links between different conceptual domains (for example social group, gender, space, time, age, seasons, food, cosmology, agriculture, animals, political power, etc.) is much more elaborate and extensive than is typical of contemporary Western societies. This has given rise to a distinction between two major modes of culturally organized thought – the *analytic* (exemplified in modern Western scientific thought), and the *analogical* or *correlative* (exemplified in many traditional societies, humoral medical theories, and classical Chinese science, amongst many other examples) (Douglas, 2000). The accounts of these forms of thought developed by historians and social anthropologists can be taken as idealized 'extrapersonal' models. Hence, the question arises of how these extrapersonal conceptual structures are interpreted and internalized by intrapersonal processes (Strauss and Quinn, 1997, and see below).

Taken together, these points suggest that even if species-level explanations identify constraints on conceptual processing, they are insufficient to *differentially* explain encultured beliefs, religious or otherwise. Rather, a model is needed which can address the questions of how group and individual-specific processes organize concepts into what Quine and Ullian termed 'webs of belief' (see Bell *et al.*, 2003), and invest such related sets of concepts and propositions with a sense of plausibility and reality.

Neoassociationist models of belief

These issues are addressed by an alternative form of cognitive anthropology that has developed in the United States, out of what was formerly known as 'psychological anthropology' (Strauss and Quinn, 1997). Recent work in this tradition has applied schema theory and connectionist accounts of learning to model cultural conditioning (Strauss and Quinn, 1997).

Schemata are 'learned, internalized patterns of thought-feeling that mediate both the interpretation of ongoing experience and the reconstruction of memories' (Strauss, 1997); they comprise 'networks of strongly connected cognitive elements that represent the generic concepts stored in memory' (Strauss and Quinn, 1997, p. 6). Cultural schemata (or cultural models) are those schemata that are widely distributed in a population, such that a '*cultural meaning* is the typical (frequently recurring and widely shared aspects of the) interpretation of some object or event evoked in people as a result of their similar life experiences' (Strauss and Quinn, 1997). On this basis, the generation of cultural beliefs would be analogous to the generation of cultural meanings.

Cultural schemata are acquired by the interaction of intrapersonal learning processes with structured regularities in the extrapersonal environment; as Strauss and Quinn put it, ' "culture" is merely a name for *all* of the learned schemas that are shared by some people, as well as all of the diverse things from which these schemas are learned' (Strauss and Quinn, 1997, p. 38). Cultural schemata 'range from highly concrete and specific constructs for things like spoons and left-turns to high-level schemas for things like love, success, authority, pollution, and the like' (D'Andrade, 1997, p. 34). Schemas show hierarchical organization, so that high-level schemas (e.g. for love or success) can instigate recruitment of lower level schemas (e.g. for joining a dating service or attending a job fair) (Strauss, 1997, p. 3).

This schema-based approach to cognitive anthropology contrasts with Sperber and Boyer's approach by its use of connectionist models of learning, rather than modularity theory. Instead of evolved conceptual dispositions and inferential biases, connectionist modelling is a form of neoassociationism: knowledge is built up by learning associations (positive or negative correlations) among the features of a number of specific cases, rather than following innate or acquired rules (Strauss and Quinn, 1997, p. 53). The developing schema begins with weights of zero or small connection weights between units in the context of a general-purpose learning algorithm, with connectional strengths modified by environmental inputs; nevertheless, the possibility of species-typical initial weights on networks is acknowledged (Strauss and Quinn, 1997). This unconscious learning is supplemented by explicit instruction and internalized 'cognitive artefacts', such as proverbs, rules of etiquette, and memorized multiplication tables (Strauss and Quinn, 1997). Schema theorists also emphasize the role of emotion in learning, arguing that emotional arousal contributes to associative learning, making some schemas more durable, including those learned early in life (Strauss and Quinn, 1997, p. 89). While schema theory is similar to modularity theory in so far as most information processing is viewed as unconscious and automatic, its emphasis on plasticity of learning gives more scope for relating the processing activities of different schemata through its models of hierarchical and implicational associative linkages between models. As such, it potentially provides a way of modelling how processing of counterintuitive concepts, for example, might be incorporated into superordinate knowledge structures.

Schema theory has been applied to the study of cultural domains such as marriage, romance, parenthood, and employment, rather than illness *per se* (Strauss, 1997; Strauss and Quinn, 1997). Nevertheless, cultural schema theorists have recognized that anthropological descriptions of cultural concepts of illness constitute extrapersonal models that constrain intrapersonal cognition, although they have yet to apply their research methods to study how these extrapersonal models of illness are internalized (Quinn, 1997, p. 211). By contrast, medical anthropologists have conducted extensive field studies using similar kinds of discourse analysis. For example research on illness narratives and explanatory models has elicited local understandings of illness and its treatment (Good, 1995; Kleinman, 1988a, 1988b; Deeley, 1999).

Good's research on local understandings of 'fainting' in Turkey is relevant to the question of how cultural schemata constitute superordinate structures within which specific kinds of conceptual processing – such as reasoning about supernatural causation – occurs (Good, 1995). Good and co-workers found that epilepsy belonged to a larger cultural domain of fainting, and that there were five major narrative types that 'emplotted' fainting episodes in characteristic ways. The commonest plot was of fainting beginning with an emotional trauma such as fright or loss, followed by a quest for cure. A second plot type was of fainting beginning with childhood fever or injury, often linked to a theme of maternal remorse for failing to protect the child. A third type was more medicalized, focusing on sudden unexplained onset, tests, and physiology. A fourth type placed epilepsy in the context of lifetimes of sadness and poverty, linking onset to life tragedies, and was not associated with extensive care seeking. Finally, in some narratives seizure onset was attributed to the evil eye, or to *jinn*, and included visits to religious shrines and healers (Good, 1995, p. 147f).

Narratives would predominantly be of one type, but would often combine features of others. It was typical for multiple interpretations and a 'network of perspectives' about an illness to develop within a family. Good argued that the discursive practices surrounding chronic illness maintain its openness to the possibility of final explanation and cure, and that the narrators of stories about chronic or relapsing illness are always 'in the middle' of the story. Overall, the narratives served to evaluate potential causes of seizures or fainting, establish coherent relationships between a number of significant life experiences, and anticipate the probable course of illness and potential sources of help or cure (Good, 1995, p. 148).

Good's research can be regarded as a delineation of widely distributed schemata that pattern local understandings of the cultural domain of fainting. Note that interpretations of the actions of the evil eye or *jinn* are located within a wider semantic network that constrains the use of those concepts. Hence, this narratological approach can be taken as evidence for the point made against Boyer's model, that processing of supernatural concepts as *beliefs* does not occur independently of locally acquired knowledge structures.

Belief and the sense of the real

Modularity and schema theories both presuppose a capacity for ideas to achieve the cognitive status of 'beliefs' – to be regarded as not merely notional, but *real*. The social processes by which a relatively small subset of possible ideas become tagged as real has been a major focus of the Durkeimian tradition, which views cultural practices as ways of investing key cultural ideas and values with a heightened sense of reality and authority:

> humans who participate collectively in magico-religious ritual performances do so precisely in order to instil belief in fictional 'other worlds'. Representations of such fictions are more than epiphenomenal; they are central in securing cognitive acknowledgement of and allegiance to the contractual intangibles underpinning cooperation in human social groups
>
> (Dunbar *et al.*, 1999, p. 6).

While the description of religious ideas as 'fictions' is more dismissively reductionist in its tone than most anthropological writing on ritual, the perspective has nevertheless been widespread (Shweder, 1997). Some social anthropologists have turned to neurobiology to identify the intrapersonal mechanisms that may mediate this social evocation of belief. In pioneering work, Victor Turner argued that the sensory components of cultural displays associatively linked strong affect and motivations to their ideological themes (Turner, 1967, 1983). More recently, Whitehouse proposed that different kinds of ritual performance evoke different kinds of memory formation (Whitehouse, 2000). Low frequency, high arousal life-crisis rituals (prominent in smaller scale 'traditional' societies) use intense sensory stimulation to generate heightened emotional states and episodic memory formation; while high-frequency, low arousal religious ceremonies (such as the Catholic mass) typically present doctrinal information, promoting semantic memory formation (Whitehouse, 2000). Nevertheless, regular worship may combine elements of 'high arousal' and 'doctrinal' teachings, such as the incorporation of healing ceremonies, speaking in tongues, and exorcism into Sunday services in evangelical Christianity or Pentecostalism in the UK. These heightened personal or vicarious experiences may be internalized as episodic memories that are recalled, interpreted, and cited as evidence of the doctrinal claims made within the religion.

Recent developments in cognitive neuroscience and neuropsychiatry can illuminate these social processes by which concepts become invested with a sense of reality. Deeley (2004) has proposed that the neurocognitive systems that 'tag' representations as real should be treated as potentially dissociable from those that invest them with emotional and motivational associations. Nevertheless, the two systems are likely to be closely integrated in development and on-line cognition. These systems – both of which are envisaged as contributing to belief formation – are modulated by two kinds of stimuli that are brought together in cultural displays such as ceremonial rituals. These are: (1) a 'sensory' route that works through the orchestration of reinforcing social-emotional signals and other stimuli (for example chanting, drumming, dancing, masks, bright colours, special foods, etc.); and (2) a 'cognitive-symbolic' route that involves presentation of perplexing but associatively suggestive verbal and non-verbal symbols. This engages a predominantly right-hemispheric semantic processing strategy to interpret what is authoratatively presented as real, if only partially understood. In this model, both components interact to promote heightened states of emotion and arousal, including activation of the mesolimbic dopamine system, which is viewed as playing a key role in 'tagging' mental representations as *real* (as distinct from merely emotive). Hence, cultural displays such as rituals modulate the activity of this system to promote the epistemic stance of 'belief' towards key representations. In phenomenological terms, participation in arousing cultural displays is experienced as intensely emotional, with loosely associative but salient semantic associations in which pattern-recognition and a sense of reality are heightened (Deeley 2004). As Knight put it, 'the gods and spirits, normally invisible, must be experienced at least periodically as more real than reality itself' (Knight, 1999, p. 230; see also Kapur, 2003 for the role of mesolimbic dopamine systems, and Brugger, 2001 for the relations between cognitive style and hemispheric predominance).

Medical training and the inculcation of belief

Ceremonial rituals represent one of many kinds of culturally organized techniques for expressing and inculcating key concepts, values, and dispositions. Specialized educational institutions have also been created to transmit beliefs and values, of which medical schools are a prime example. Good and colleagues conducted an ethnographic study of medical education at Harvard medical school, over 4 years in the mid-1980s, to examine the processes by which the distinctive body of concepts, assumptions, values, and competences of doctors are reproduced (Good, 1995).

The research focused on 'practices and experiences common to students . . . , many of which are viewed as so ordinary as to merit little attention' (Good, 1995, p. 66). On this basis, Good argued that 'entry into the world of medicine is accomplished not only by learning the language and knowledge base of medicine, but by learning quite fundamental practices through which medical practitioners engage and formulate reality in a specifically "medical" way. These include specialized ways of "seeing", "writing", and "speaking" ' (Good, 1995, p. 71).

A new kind of 'seeing' is learned in the preclinical years, when much time is spent teaching skills of perceptual discrimination in conjunction with factual knowledge through dissection of the cadaver: 'anatomy required a training of the eyes, to see structure where none was obvious', so that 'veins and arteries, nerves, lymphatic vessels, and connective tissue were largely indistinguishable from one another until weeks into gross anatomy' (Good, 1995, p. 73). This gross anatomical cognitive–perceptual knowledge is integrated with microscopy of various kinds: 'modern imaging techniques give a powerful sense of authority to biological reality. Look in the microscope, you can see it. Electron microscopy reveals histological concepts as literal' (Good, 1995, p. 74).

Good suggests that 'if mathematical relationships govern astronomy or physics, three-dimensional shapes remain central in biology' (Good, 1995, p. 73), and the different scales at which three-dimensional shapes are learned are organized by a pervasive schema. This schema identifies successive layers of biological reality in a movement from the macroscopic to the microscopic level. For example slide shows in lectures typically followed a format in which a slide about the epidemiology of disease would be followed by successive slides of a patient, a pathological specimen, a low magnification of cell structure, and finally by an electron micrograph.

This schema was evident in the choice of prototypic diseases. For example, 'myaesthenia gravis, a quite rare neurological disorder, has a central place in neurobiology courses, because it is accounted for by a disorder of antibodies to the acetylcholine receptor. Diseases with known, specific mechanisms are taught as prototypes. The message is clear. The architecture of knowledge is in place; we only need to fill in the missing structural links' (Good, 1995, p. 76).

Hence, 'the first two years of medical education provide a powerful interpretation of reality, anchored in the experience of the student. Surface phenomena of signs, symptoms and experience are shown to be understandable with reference to underlying mechanisms at an ontologically prior level. Even broadly incorporative biopsychosocial models, articulated in the language of systems theory, represent biology at the center, social relations outward at the periphery' (Good, 1995, p. 76).

Good's analysis of a distinctive biomedical ontology and epistemology recalls the distinction between 'analytic' and 'correlative' thought described above. Western science relies on analogies as do other kinds of world-view, but the use of analogy in Western science tends to be restricted to specific domains of explanation, and tightly bound to experimental approaches – for example the analogy of billiard balls to work out the kinetic theory of gases (Douglas, 2000). Correlative thinking, by contrast, maps extensive analogical relations and equivalences between different conceptual domains (gender, space, time, food, animals, for example) (Douglas, 2000). What is striking about Good's account of biomedicine, though, is how an 'analytic' discipline (governed by experimental procedures and tightly controlled analogies) allows such extensive ontological correspondences to be posited between different 'levels' of reality. In that respect, the biomedical model resembles a correlative system of knowledge, although the links between levels are modelled in mechanistic terms. In Good's view, biomedicine has produced a reversal of the hierarchical ordering of the world from material to divine: 'unlike in the Platonic, medieval and renaissance view, . . . ultimacy resides in depth, downward to levels that generate surface phenomena. And such deeper structures are not social or divine but ever more fundamental orders of material reality' (Good, 1995, p. 75). Good comments on the bias this introduces into medical understandings of the complex human phenomena of illness and disease, where attention and resources tend to be invested into researching and manipulating small scale material phenomena such as genes and antibodies, over, say, social or psychological processes.

During clinical training, Good argues that this conceptual structure shapes the distinctive ways in which medical students learn to talk and write about patients. Students learn to formulate a case in terms of evidence for and against a diagnosis; as a student commented, 'of course the real world doesn't lend itself to that, so you distort the real world a little bit to make it fit that nice pattern' (Good, 1995, p. 77). As another student commented, 'they don't want to hear the story of the person. They want to hear the edited version' (Good, 1995, p. 77). Similarly, the skill of writing in notes 'provides a structure of relevance that justifies the systematic discounting of the patient's narrative. It organizes the patient as a document, a project to be worked on' (Good, 1995, p. 78).

Good presents his analysis of medical training not as a critique, but as an attempt to understand an intensive form of socialization, in which a formulation of 'sickness from a materialist and individualizing perspective' is inculcated, in conjunction with an immense body of knowledge and skills (Good, 1995, p. 83). He points out that as the skills are internalized, clinicians have more scope to integrate a more person-focused concern in their practice, at least ideally. He also argues that biomedicine, despite its materialist conception of illness, is also deeply fused with moral conceptions and 'soteriological' issues (that is, referring to suffering and salvation), and at times these dimensions of illness 'erupt as the central issues of medical practice' (Good, 1995, p. 67; see Good, 1995, p. 83 ff for examples such as the emphasis on protecting or prolonging 'life' in the allocation of medical resources and clinical priorities).

Further, it is clear from his account that 'belief' – understood in Sperber's sense as 'a disposition to express, assent to, or otherwise act in accordance with some proposition' (Sperber, 1996), is just one aspect of the substantial reorganization of cognition and skills that occurs during medical training. While he does not discuss his findings in cognitive terms, his analysis suggests that many cognitive processes are brought into integrated functional relationships to support the distinctive kinds of interpretations, self-representation, and practice that are typical of medicine – these would include functions such as perceptual expertise, attention, planning, semantic and procedural memory, as well as a general demeanour and style involving distinctive social scripts, facial expressions, speech prosody, and pragamatics. Social approval and disapproval from teachers and clinicians, ranging from praise to humiliation, are powerful means of motivating effort and conformity. These emotive experiences are associated with their own episodic memories. Further, strong emotions and changes in self-schemata are also evoked by the way in which social taboos about intimate contact with the dead and the living are collectively broken in a socially sanctioned way; as one female student commented, 'we handle cadavers, have feces lab where we examine our own feces, go to [a mental hospital where we get locked up with] screaming patients. These are total experiences, like an occult thing or a boot camp' (Good, 1995, p. 65). Hence, Good's analysis of medical training reinforces the point that the acquisition of beliefs must be understood in the context of social constraints on other aspects of cognition, experience, and behaviour.

Conclusion

In this chapter I have reviewed contributions of cognitive anthropology to understanding 'the power of belief', supplementing the accounts with reference to social and medical anthropology where appropriate. I have attempted to show that there is considerable scope for dialogue between anthropology and cognitive science, and that group level (cultural) processes contribute to cognition, in addition to species-level and within-group constraints. An ongoing challenge will be to continue to develop ways of integrating the experimental approach of cognitive science with the anthropological tradition of describing and interpreting the complex social and informational environments that human beings inhabit (Sperber and Hirschfeld, 2001). Further, while cognitive neuroscience has made substantial progress through devising methods to isolate and examine discrete functions such as 'selective attention' or 'episodic memory', anthropological accounts of mind and behaviour draw attention to the theoretical challenge of demon-strating how fractionated cognitive processes, including those underlying beliefs, are functionally integrated to support the kinds of locally coherent and meaningful participation in diverse social contexts that is typical of human beings (Deeley, 1999).

References

Barrett JL (2000). Exploring the natural foundations of religion. *Trends in Cognitive Sciences*, **4**, 29–34.

Barrett JL and Keil FC (1996). Conceptualizing a nonnatural entity: anthropomorphism in God concepts. *Cognitive Psychology*, **31**, 219–247.

Bell V, Halligan P and Ellis H (2003). Beliefs about delusions. *Psychologist*, **16**, 418–423.

Bowker J (1987). *Licensed insanities: religions and belief in God in the contemporary world.* London: Dartman, Longman, and Todd.

Boyer P (2000). Evolution of the modern mind and the origins of culture: religious concepts as a limiting case. In: PC Carruthers and A Chamberlain, eds. *Evolution and the human mind: modularity, language and meta-cognition.* Cambridge: Cambridge University Press, pp. 93–112.

Boyer P (2002). *Religion explained.* Vintage.

Boyer P (2003). Religious thought and behaviour as by-products of brain function. *Trends in Cognitive Sciences*, **7**, 110–124.

Boyer P and Ramble C (2001). Cognitive templates for religious concepts: cross-cultural evidence for recall of counter-intuitive representations. *Cognitive Science*, **25**, 535–564.

Brugger P (2001). From haunted brain to haunted science: a cognitive neuroscience view of paranormal and pseudoscientific thought. In: JL Houran and RJ Lange, eds. *Hauntings and poltergeists: multidisciplinary perspectives.* Jefferson, NC: McFarland, pp. 195–213.

D'Andrade R (1997). Schemas and motivation. In: R D'Andrade and C Strauss, eds. *Human motives and cultural models*, Cambridge: Cambridge University Press, pp. 23–44.

Dawkins R (1976). *The selfish gene.* New York: Oxford University Press.

Deeley PQ (1999). Medicine, psychiatry, and the ecology of mind. *Philosophy, Psychiatry, and Psychology*, **6**, 109–124.

Deeley PQ (2000). Differences in ritual and culture. In: C Kaye, ed. *Transcultural psychiatry: working with difference.* London: Jessica Kingsley Publications.

Deeley PQ (2004). The religious brain: turning ideas into convictions. *Anthropology and Medicine*, Vol II, 3, 245–267.

Douglas M (2000). *Leviticus as literature.* Oxford: Oxford University Press.

Dunbar R, Knight C and Power C, eds (1999). *The evolution of culture.* Edinburgh: Edinburgh University Press.

Durham W (1991). *Coevolution: genes, culture, and human diversity.* Stanford: Stanford University Press.

Good B (1995). *Medicine, rationality and experience: an anthropological perspective.* Cambridge: Cambridge University Press.

Guthrie S (1980). A cognitive theory of religion. *Current Anthropology*, **21**, 181–203.

Hollis M and Lukes S (1982). *Rationality and relativism.* Oxford: Basil Blackwell.

Kapur S (2003). Psychosis as a state of aberrant salience: a framework for linking biology, phenomenology, and pharmacology in schizophrenia. *American Journal of Psychiatry*, **160**, 13–23.

Kleinman A (1988a). *Rethinking psychiatry: from cultural category to personal experience.* New York: Free Press.

Kleinman A (1988b). *The illness narratives: suffering, healing and the human condition.* New York: Basic Books.

Knight C (1999). Sex and language as pretend play. In: R Dunbar, C Knight and C Power, eds. *The evolution of culture.* Edinburgh: Edinburgh University Press.

Leslie C and Young A (1992). *Paths to Asian medical knowledge.* Berkeley, Los Angeles, Oxford: University of California Press.

Littlewood R (2002). *Pathologies of the West: an anthropology of mental illness in Europe and America.* London: Continuum.

Littlewood R and Lipsedge M (1989). *Aliens and alienists: ethnic minorities and psychiatrists.* London: Unwin-Hyman.

Macdonald M, ed. (1990). *Witchcraft and Hysteria in Elizabethan London.* London, New York: Tavistock/Routledge.

Ortner SB (1984). Theory in anthropology since the sixties. *Comparative Studies in Society and History,* **26,** 126 –125.

Quinn N (1997). The motivational force of self-understanding: evidence from wives' inner conflicts. In: R D'Andrade and C Strauss, eds. *Human motives and cultural models,* Cambridge: Cambridge University Press, pp. 90–126.

Shweder RA (1997). Ghost busters in anthropology. In: R D'Andrade and C Strauss, eds. *Human motives and cultural models,* Cambridge: Cambridge University Press, pp. 45–57.

Sperber D (1996). *Explaining culture.* Oxford: Blackwell.

Sperber D and Hirschfeld L (2001). Culture, cognition, and evolution. In: RA Wilson and FC Keil, eds. *The MIT encyclopedia of the cognitive sciences,* pp. cxi–cxxxii. Cambridge, Massachuritts, London, England: MIT Press.

Strauss C (1997). Models and motives. In: R D'Andrade and C Strauss, eds. *Human motives and cultural models,* Cambridge University Press. pp. 1–20.

Strauss C and Quinn N (1997). *A cognitive theory of cultural meaning.* Cambridge: Cambridge University Press.

Turner V (1967). *The forest of symbols.* Ithaca and London: Cornell University Press.

Turner V (1983). Body, brain, and culture. *Zygon,* **18,** 221–245.

Whitehouse H (2000). *Arguments and icons: divergent modes of religiosity.* Oxford: Oxford University Press.

Chapter 4

Placebo: the role of expectancies in the generation and alleviation of illness

Irving Kirsch

Introduction

Placebo has been defined as the most frequently studied of all medical treatments. More seriously, it is often characterized as a 'non-specific' treatment. But what does it mean to say that a treatment is non-specific? It might mean that the specific characteristics of the treatment are unrelated to the effects of the treatment. But this is not true of placebos. As shown below, the effects of a placebo vary as a function of its colour, name, dose, and mode of administration. Also, the chemical composition of the placebo can make a difference. Not all placebos are inert. There are also active placebos, which are substances that mimic some of the side-effects of a drug but do not have a pharmacological effect on the condition being treated. The therapeutic benefits of active placebos may be greater than those of inert placebos, at least in the treatment of depression (Greenberg and Fisher, 1989; Moncrieff *et al.*, 2001).

A second potential meaning of the term 'non-specific' is that the treatment affects a wide variety of conditions, rather than just one or two specific conditions. This certainly is true of placebos. Included among the conditions and responses that placebos have been shown to affect are tension, anxiety, alertness, hypertension, depression, pain, sexual arousal, asthma, nausea, vomiting, blood pressure, heart rate, ulcers, angina, rheumatoid arthritis, Parkinson's disease, contact dermatitis, warts, and infections (Kirsch, 1990, 1999). But if placebos are non-specific in this sense of the term, so are aspirin and morphine.

The current characterization of placebo as a non-specific treatment may be due to an historical accident. According to the Oxford English Dictionary (2nd edition, 1989), the term *specific* was first used in a medical context in the 17th century as a noun denoting a physical substance used as a remedy.

Thus, any treatment that is not a physical substance (psychotherapy, for example) is a non-specific, regardless of how effective it is.

What, then, is a placebo? It is a physical substance or procedure presented as having physical properties that, in fact, it does not have. Efforts have been made to extend the placebo concept to psychological treatments (e.g. Stewart-Williams and Podd, in press), but others have argued that this extension is untenable (Kirsch, 1978, 2004, in press). In this chapter, I review evidence indicating the power of placebos to affect physical and emotional responses, some of the factors that influence the placebo effect, and the clinical implications of these data.

The power of placebo

A review in the *New England Journal of Medicine* questioned the belief that placebos can produce powerful effects. Hróbjartsson and Gøtzsche (2001) reported a meta-analysis in which they purported to compare the placebo effect to no treatment. Their results indicated a small but significant placebo effect in studies reporting continuous outcome scores and a non-significant effect in studies reporting dichotomous outcomes. However, there is good reason to believe that this is a gross underestimate of the placebo effect.

Hróbjartsson and Gøtzsche (2001) analyzed clinical trials of treatments for a motley collection of disorders, including the common cold, alcohol abuse, smoking, poor oral hygiene, herpes simplex infection, infertility, mental retardation, marital discord, faecal soiling, Alzheimer's disease, carpal tunnel syndrome, and 'undiagnosed ailments.' The 'placebos' in these clinical trials were not limited to conventional pill placebos, but instead included relaxation (classified as a treatment in some of the studies and as a placebo in others); leisure reading; answering questions about hobbies, newspapers, magazines, favourite foods and favourite sports teams; and talking about daily events, family activities, football, vacation activities, pets, hobbies, books, movies, and television shows. Not surprisingly, the most reliable finding in the Hróbjartsson and Gøtzsche (2001) meta-analysis was that there was substantial and significant heterogeneity in the outcomes produced by placebo. In other words, either some placebos were significantly more effective than others, some disorders were more amenable to placebo treatment than others, or both. In other words, the placebo is specific, not non-specific! This, in itself, validates the existence of a placebo effect. One placebo cannot be more effective than another unless placebos are capable of producing an effect.

In fact, there are considerable data indicating placebo effects that are powerful and long lasting. Some of the studies indicating particularly strong placebo effects are reviewed in this section.

Parkinson's disease

Placebos have been found to produce a strong curative effect on Parkinson's disease (Fuente-Fernández et al., 2002). Lasting effects (up to 18 months) have been observed on all objective measures of motor performance and neuroimaging studies indicate that they are associated with activation of the nigrostriatal dopaminergic pathway, leading to the release of dopamine in the striatum. This can be regarded as a very specific effect, in as much as Parkinson's disease is produced by a deficiency of dopamine. The placebo-induced biochemical effect in patients with Parkinson's disease equals that of the active drug apomorphine.

Rheumatoid arthritis

Traut and Passarelli (1957) reported a study of the effect of placebo on rheumatoid arthritis. An improvement rate of 50 per cent was observed following administration of placebo pills. Those showing no improvement following the pills were then given injections of the placebo. This brought the improvement rate up to 82 per cent and lasted until the study was discontinued 30 months later. Specificity of this placebo effect was shown by the finding that improvement was greatest when the site of the injection was close to the affected part of the body.

Asthma

Asthmatic patients exhibit bronchoconstriction after inhaling a placebo described as a bronchoconstrictor and brochodilation after inhaling a placebo described as a bronchodilator (Sodergren and Hyland, 1999). These placebo affects are about two-thirds the magnitude of the active agents and when people are misinformed about *whether* agent is a bronchoconstrictor or bronchodilator, this misinformation cuts the pharmacological effect in half.

Contact dermatitus

In a study reported by Ikemi and Nakagawa (1962), 13 students were touched on one arm with leaves from a harmless tree, but were told that the leaves were from a lacquer or wax tree (Japanese trees that produce effects similar to poison ivy and to which the students had reported being hypersensitive). On the other arm, the students were touched with poisonous leaves, which they were led to believe were from a harmless tree. All 13 subjects displayed a skin reaction to the harmless leaves (the placebo), but only two reacted to the poisonous leaves. Five of the students had been hypnotized before being touched with the leaves, but the results were virtually identical for hypnotized and non-hypnotized subjects.

Gastric function

A series of studies by Stewart Wolf (1950), a pioneer in the investigation of placebo effects, indicate that placebo effects can be powerful enough to reverse the effect of active drugs. One of Wolf's patients was a 28-year-old woman who was suffering from the nausea and vomiting that sometimes accompanies the early stages of pregnancy. Wolf gave her ipecac, a drug that interrupts normal gastric contractions, thereby inducing vomiting and nausea. Although ipecac is commonly used to induce vomiting when toxic substances have been swallowed, Wolf misinformed his patient that it was a medicine which would alleviate her nausea. Prior to taking ipecac, the patient displayed an absence of gastric contractions. Within 20 minutes after ingesting the drug, normal gastric contractions resumed and the nausea ended.

Wolf (1950) conducted a similar experiment on another patient suffering from nausea associated with recurrent interruptions of gastric contractions. When administered orally without counteracting instructions, ipecac predictably induced nausea and vomiting. However, when the same dosage was administered in disguised form and was accompanied by misinformation about its effects, it produced a resumption of normal contractile activity and the nausea disappeared.

The best known of Wolf's demonstrations of placebo effects on gastric function involved 'Tom,' whose enlarged gastric fistula made it possible to directly observe his gastric mucous membrane. Because of his condition, Tom was the subject of more than 100 experiments on the effects of various drugs. One of these was prostigmine, a drug that produces gastric hyperfunction, abdominal cramps, and diarrhoea. These effects were later reproduced by inert placebos and also by atropine sulfate, which typically inhibits gastric function (Wolf, 1950). In another experiment, Tom was observed following 13 administrations of a placebo and during 13 control trials in which no substance had been given to him (Abbot *et al.*, 1952). Placebo administration resulted in a 33 per cent decrease in gastric acid secretion, as compared to an 18 per cent decrease during control trials.

Sexual dysfunction

Placebo effects are mediated by response expectancy (Kirsch, 1985, 1999; Stewart-Williams and Podd, in press). The clinical significance of expectancy effects on sexual arousal have been demonstrated in an impressive series of studies by Eileen Palace (1999) and her colleagues. In one of these studies, Palace used false biofeedback of vaginal blood volume (VBV) during exposure to erotic stimuli to test her hypothesis that sexual response expectancies alter sexual response. She reported that false VBV feedback indicating arousal increased actual VBV in 100 per cent of sexually dysfunctional women and the increase in actual response occurred within 30 seconds of the expectation of an increase, thus providing strong evidence for the causal role of expectancy.

Pain and anxiety

The effects of placebos on pain and anxiety have been well established (Price and Barrell, 1999; Schoenberger, 1999). Recently, a methodology has been developed for assessing the placebo effect without the use of placebos and has been applied to assessing the placebo component of pharmacological treatment of pain and anxiety (Benedetti *et al.*, 2003). Participants give permission to receive a medication with or without foreknowledge of the onset of administration. Medication is subsequently administered intravenously, in some cases with the patient's knowledge and in other cases without any signal. Using this methodology, Benedetti and colleagues found that a substantial proportion of the effects of morphine on pain is a placebo effect. In addition, they reported that the effect of diazepam on postoperative anxiety was entirely a placebo effect, because hidden infusions of diazepam were totally ineffective in reducing postoperative anxiety.

Depression

A meta-analysis of published studies indicated a change of 1.16 standard deviations on measures of depression following administration of placebo antidepressants, compared to a change of 0.37 standard deviations among untreated controls (Kirsch and Sapirstein, 1998). These data indicate a placebo effect size of 0.79 standard deviations. This is a powerful effect by any standard, but it may be an underestimate. Most clinical trials of antidepressant medication fail to show a significant difference between drug and placebo (Kirsch *et al.*, 2002). Almost all of the studies showing a significant difference have been published, whereas most of those failing to find a difference have been withheld from publication (Melander *et al.*, 2003), thus producing the illusion of a strong antidepressant drug effect. In fact, the placebo effect of antidepressant medication appears to be substantially greater than the pharmacological effect.

There is yet another reason for suspecting that the data reported by Kirsch and Sapirstein (1998) underestimate the placebo effect on depression. Included in the data base they analyzed were four medications (amylobarbitone, lithium, liothyronine, and adinazolam) that are not antidepressants. The change produced by these active placebos (1.69 SDs) was greater than that of inert placebos and as great as that observed in patients given selective serotonin reuptake inhibitors (SSRIs) (1.68 SDs) and tricyclics (1.52 SDs). This suggests that the response to antidepressant medication may be entirely a placebo response.

Why do active placebos produce stronger effects on depression than inert placebos? The key may be the breaking of blind by patients randomized to the drug condition in conventional clinical trials. In double-blind trials of antidepressant medication, most patients (especially those assigned to the drug condition) and their physicians break the blind and successfully deduce the condition to which they have been assigned (Rabkin *et al.*, 1986). This appears to be due to the greater occurrence of side-effects in the drug condition (Greenberg and Fisher, 1989). In any case, knowing that one has been assigned to the drug condition is likely to enhance the placebo effect, whereas knowledge of assignment to the placebo group ought to decrease its effect. Thus, at least part (and maybe all) of the small difference between drug and placebo may be an enhanced placebo effect due to the breaking of blind.

Factors affecting the placebo response

Colour

The colour of a placebo can influence its effects. When administered without information about whether they are stimulants or depressives, blue placebo pills produce depressant effects, whereas red placebos induce stimulant effects (Blackwell *et al.*, 1972). Patients report falling asleep significantly more quickly and sleeping longer after taking a blue capsule than after taking an orange capsule (Luchelli *et al.*, 1978). Red placebos are more effective pain relievers than white, blue, or green placebos (Huskisson, 1974; Nagao *et al.*, 1968).

Label

The magnitude of the placebo effect varies with the strength of the treatment it is replacing. Placebo morphine is more effective than propoxyphene, which, in turn, is more effective than aspirin (Evans, 1974). Placebos bearing a well-known brand name are more effective than those administered without the brand name (Branthwaite and Cooper, 1981). This, of course, must be the case. Were it not, it is difficult to fathom how pharmaceutical companies could succeed in selling brand name drugs for which generic equivalents are available at lower prices. Finally, simply switching from one placebo to another can enhance the placebo effect (Rickels *et al.*, 1964). This is particularly important given the experience of clinicians who prescribe antidepressants. Patients who fail to respond to a particular antidepressant are often switched to another, following which they sometimes improve. The phenomenon is sometimes interpreted as evidence of the efficacy of antidepressants (Hollon *et al.*, 2002). Instead, it might be the same phenomena observed by Rickels *et al.* (1964), that is a benefit derived from the perception that a different medication is being tried.

Dose

Placebo effects are dose dependent. Two pills are more effective than one (Rickels *et al.*, 1970) and four are more effective than two (de Craen *et al.* 1999). Similarly, two cups of coffee increase subjective and physiological indices of arousal more than one, even if (unknown to the recipient) the coffee is decaffeinated (Kirsch and Weixel, 1988).

Mode of administration

The way in which the placebo is administered can also make a difference. Placebo capsules are more effective than placebo pills (Hussain and Ahad, 1970) and placebo injections are more effective than orally administered placebos (de Craen *et al.*, 2000). Surgery may be the most effective method of administering a placebo.

Placebo surgery involves making an incision, but then not performing the surgical procedure. The first trials of surgical procedures that including sham surgery as a control procedure appears to have been those testing mammary ligation in the treatment of angina (Cobb *et al.*, 1959; Dimond *et al.*, 1960). Mammary ligation had been used as a treatment for angina since the 1940s and was considered exceptionally effective. Across the two controlled trials, 73 per cent of the patients receiving mammary ligation showed substantial improvement. The improvement rate with placebo surgery was 83 per cent. Needless to say, mammary ligation is no longer used as a treatment for angina.

More recently, sham surgery has been used in the evaluation of treatments for osteoarthritis of the knee (Moseley *et al.*, 2002) and Parkinson's disease (Freed *et al.*, 2001; Watts *et al.*, 2001). Moseley *et al.* (2002) reported the results of a large (180 patients) placebo-controlled clinical trial evaluating the effects arthroscopic surgery on pain and mobility in patients with osteoarthritis. In the placebo group, incisions were made and the surgery was simulated, but the arthroscope was not inserted. In previous uncontrolled studies, response rates ranging from 44 to 88 per cent had been reported for this procedure. In Moseley *et al.*'s study, the effects of the surgery were duplicated by the sham surgery. In fact, the only significant differences between real and placebo surgery was that patients given the sham treatment reported less pain and better physical functioning 2 weeks after the procedure. At the final assessment

2 years later, these differences had disappeared and there were no longer any significant differences between real and placebo surgery. Why did the short-term differences favour placebo? The authors speculated that this may have been due to the fact that patients undergoing the sham procedure were spared the surgical trauma.

Real and placebo surgery in the treatment of Parkinson's disease have been compared in two clinical trials. Freed *et al.* (2001) used sham surgery to evaluate implantation of human embryonic dopamine neurons into the brains of patients with Parkinson's disease. Watts *et al.* (2001) used placebo surgery to evaluate the effects of pocine fetal transplants. Sham surgery consisted of drilling holes in the skull without penetrating the dura. In the Freed *et al.* study, real surgery produced a significant benefit compared to placebo surgery, but only among younger patients. In the Watts *et al.* study, there was no difference between real and placebo surgery. Both produced substantial improvement lasting more than 18 months.

Questions are often raised about the efficacy of using placebo controls in clinical trials. How can one justify giving patients a sham treatment when an effective alternative may be available? This concern seems even more acute in surgery. How can one justify cutting people open and sewing them up again without therapeutic benefit? Of course, there often is therapeutic benefit from the use of placebo and it may be as great as that provided by the surgery or medication that is being investigated. So if one can raise ethical questions about the administration of a placebo, similar questions can be raised about the administration of a treatment that has not yet been proven effective. But there is a more compelling argument to be made for the use of placebos, including surgical placebos, in clinical trials. Suppose that placebo surgery had not been used in a controlled test of mammary ligation. In that case, we would never have learned that the benefits of this surgical procedure are entirely due to the placebo effect. Over the years, placebo surgery would have been performed on hundreds of thousands of patients, without the patients or their physicians ever knowing that the surgery was really a placebo. Given this consequence, it might be considered unethical to *not* do a placebo controlled trial if there is a reasonable possibility that the benefits of a treatment are placebo effects.

Adherence

Finally, one needs to take the placebo in order for it to have an effect. This was dramatically illustrated in a 5-year study of the effects of the cholesterol-lowering medication clofibrate on the mortality rates of nearly 4000 postmyocardial infarction patients (Coronary Drug Project Group, 1980). The main finding was a spectacular lack of success for the active medication.

Twenty per cent of the patients given clofibrate died within the 5-year period, compared to 21 per cent of those given placebo. One of the problems in evaluating a medication is the fact that many people who are given a medication fail to take it as prescribed. To check for the impact of lack of adherence, the researchers divided the sample into those who had taken at least 80 per cent of the pill that were prescribed (good adherers) and those who had taken less than 80 per cent (poor adherers). The difference in mortality between these two groups was statistically significant. Twenty-five per cent of the poor adherers had died, compared to only 15 pr cent of the good adherers. This would seem to indicate a powerful drug effect that was being masked by poor compliance among some of the patients in the trial. However, a similar difference was found in the placebo condition: 28 per cent of the poor adherers had died, compared with 15 per cent of the good adherers. Similar effects of compliance in the placebo condition have been reported for antibiotics (Pizzo et al., 1983), beta-blockers (Gallagher et al., 1993; Horwitz et al., 1990), and antipsychotic medication (Hogarty and Goldberg, 1973).

Harnessing the placebo effect

This review reveals that placebo treatment may be effective for a wide variety of physical and psychological conditions. Compared to conventional medical treatments, it has an advantage of producing substantially fewer side-effects, although placebo-induced side-effects have also been documented (Pogge, 1963). The problem with knowingly prescribing placebos is that it requires clinicians to deceive their patients. Expectancy is only one psychological factor that can influence healing. Another is the patient's trust in the healer. But trust has to be earned. Trust that is repeatedly violated will eventually be lost. So the problem is to find ways of utilizing the placebo effect without deception.

One key to doing this is the finding that placebo and drug effects are sometimes (but not always) additive (Kirsch, 2000). In other words, positive expectations may enhance the effectiveness of an active treatment. The most recent evidence of additivity can be found in a series of studies reported by Fabrizio Benedetti and his colleagues, in which participants gave permission to receive a medication with or without foreknowledge of the onset of administration, as described above (Benedetti et al., 2003). If placebo and drug effects are additive, then expressions of confidence in an active treatment should enhance its effectiveness and indeed there are data indicating this to be the case. Blasi et al. (2001) reviewed 25 studies in which physicians attempted to influence patients' expectancies about the efficacy of the treatment. The

Prevaricain®
A genuine placebo medication

- **Tested** in more clinical trials than any other treatment.
- **Powerful**: the standard by which all other medications are tested.
- **Effective** in the treatment of thousands of ailments.
- **Safe** enough for infants, the elderly, and pregnant women.

If it's a placebo, you can believe in it!

Fig. 4.1 A possible advertisement for placebos if these were ever to be marketed.

general finding was that positive messages tend to enhance treatment outcome. Four of these studies also manipulated the warmth of the treating physician and these tended to show the strongest effects, but this factor was not looked at independently. Thus, based on the available data, expressions of confidence in a treatment can enhance the treatments effects and this may be potentiated if the message is delivered in the context of a warm and friendly atmosphere. This is a placebo effect produced without placebos and without deception.

The problem remains of what to do when an active treatment is not available or not advisable. For example antidepressant medication adds little clinical benefit to the placebo response. Specifically, the pharmaceutical company clinical trial data indicate that improvement in moderately to severely depressed patients following administration of SSRIs is approximately 10 points on the Hamilton depression scale, compared to more than 8 points improvement following administration of placebo (Kirsch *et al.*, 2002). A 10 point change on the Hamilton scale is clinically significant, as is an 8 point change, but the difference between them is not.

Fortunately, there are a number of empirically validated alternatives to medication for depressed patients. These include psychotherapy, self-help books, exercise, and herbal remedies. Still, it would be particularly efficient and cost effective if simple inert (or at least benign) placebos could be prescribed ethically. Despite my belief that they cannot, I cannot help but imagine what would happen if they could be. In particular, I envision placebo advertisements like that shown in Fig. 4.1.

References

Abbot FK, Mack M and Wolf S (1952). The action of banthine on the stomach and duodenum of man with observations of the effects of placebos. *Gastroenterology*, **20**, 249–269.

Benedetti F, Maggi G, Lopiano L, Lanotte M, Rainero I, Vighetti S and Pollo A (2003). Open versus hidden medical treatments: The patient's knowledge about a therapy affects the therapy outcome. *Prevention and Treatment,* **6**, Article 1. Available at: http://journals.apa.org/prevention/volume6/pre0060001a.html.

Blackwell B, Bloomfield SS and Buncher CR (1972). Demonstration to medical students of placebo responses and non-drug factors. *Lancet,* **19**, 1279–1282.

Blasi ZD, Harkness E, Ernst E, Georgiou A and Kleijnen J (2001). Influence of context effects on health outcomes: a systematic review. *Lancet,* **357**, 752–762.

Branthwaite A and Cooper P (1981). Analgesic effects of branding in treatment of headaches. *British Medical Journal (Clinical Research Edition),* **282**, 1576–1578.

Cobb L, Thomas GI, Dillard DH, Merendino KA and Bruce RA (1959). An evaluation of internal-mammary artery ligation by a double blind technique. *New England Journal of Medicine,* **260**, 1115–1118.

Coronary Drug Project Group (1980). Influence of adherence to treatment and response of cholesterol on mortality in the coronary drug project. *New England Journal of Medicine,* **303**, 1038–1041.

de Craen AJM, Moerman DE, Heisterkamp SH, Tytgat GNJ, Tijssen JPG and Kleijnen J (1999). Placebo effect in the treatment of duodenal ulcer. *British Journal of Clinical Pharmacology,* **48**, 853–860.

de Craen AJM, Tijssen JGP, de Gans J and Kleijnen J (2000). Placebo effect in the acute treatment of migraine: Subcutaneous placebos are better than oral placebos. *Journal of Neurology,* **247**, 183–188.

Dimond EG, Kittle CF and Crockett JE (1960). Comparison of internal mammary ligation and sham operation for angina pectoris. *American Journal of Cardiology,* **5**, 483–486.

Evans FJ (1974). The placebo response in pain reduction. In: JJ Bonica, ed. *Advances in Neurology, vol. 4, Pain,* pp. 289–296. New York: Raven.

Freed CR, Greene PE, Breeze RE, Tsai WY, DuMouchel W, Kao R, Dillon S, Winfield H, Culver S, Trojanowski JQ, Eidelberg D and Fahn S (2001). Transplantation of embryonic dopamine neurons for severe Parkinson's disease. *New England Journal of Medicine,* **344**, 710–719.

Fuente-Fernández R, Schultzer M and Stoessi AJ (2002). The placebo effect in neurological disorders. *Lancet Neurology,* **1**, 85–91.

Gallagher EJ, Viscoli CM and Horwitz RI (1993). The relationship of treatment adherence to the risk of death after myocardial infarction in women. *Journal of the American Medical Association,* **270**, 742–744.

Greenberg RP and Fisher S (1989). Examining antidepressant effectiveness: Findings, ambiguities and some vixing puzzles. In: S Fisher and RP Greenberg, eds. *The limits of biological treatments for psychological distress: Comparisons with psychotherapy and placebo,* pp. 1–37. Hillsdale, NJ: Lawrence Erlbaum.

Hogarty GE and Goldberg SC (1973). Drug and sociotherapy in the aftercare of schizophrenic patient: One-year relapse rates. *Archives of General Psychiatry,* **28**, 54–64.

Hollon SD, DeRubeis RJ, Shelton RC and Weiss B (2002). The Emperor's new drugs: effect size and moderation effects. *Prevention and Treatment.*

Horwitz RI, Viscoli CM, Berkman L, Donaldson RM, Horwitz SM, Murray CJ, Ransohoff DF and Sindelar J (1990). Treatment adherence and risk of death after myocardial infarction. *Lancet,* **336**, 542–545.

Hróbjartsson A and Gøtzsche PC (2001). An analysis of clinical trials comparing placebo with no treatment. *New England Journal of Medicine*, **344**, 1594–1602.

Huskisson E (1974). Simple analgesics for arthritis. *British Medial Journal*, **4**, 196–200.

Hussain MZ and Ahad A (1970). Tablet colour in anxiety states. *British Medical Journal*, **3**, 466.

Ikemi Y and Nakagawa S (1962). A psychosomatic study of contagious dermatitis. *Kyoshu Journal of Medical Science*, **13**, 335–350.

Kirsch I (1978). The placebo effect and the cognitive-behavioral revolution. *Cognitive Therapy and Research*, **2**, 255–264.

Kirsch I (1985). Response expectancy as a determinant of experience and behavior. *American Psychologist*, **40**, 1189–1202.

Kirsch I (1990). *Changing expectations: A key to effective psychotherapy*. Pacific Grove, CA: Brooks/Cole.

Kirsch I (1999). *How expectancies shape experience*. Washington, DC: American Psychological Association.

Kirsch I (2000). Are drug and placebo effects in depression additive? *Biological Psychiatry*, **47**, 733–735.

Kirsch I (2004). Conditioning, expectancy and the placebo effect: A comment on Stewart-Williams and Podd (2004). *Psychological Bulletin*, **130**, 341–43.

Kirsch I (2005). Placebo psychotherapy: Synonym or oxymoron? *Journal of Clinical Psychology*, **61**(7), 791–803.

Kirsch I, Moore TJ, Scoboria A and Nicholls SS (2002). The emperor's new drugs: An analysis of antidepressant medication data submitted to the FDA. *Prevention and Treatment*. Available at: http://www.journals.apa.org/prevention/volume5/pre0050023a.html.

Kirsch I and Sapirstein G (1998). Listening to Prozac but hearing placebo: A meta-analysis of antidepressant medication. *Prevention and Treatment*, **1**, Article 0002a. Available at: http://www.journals.apa.org/prevention/volume1/pre0010002a.html.

Kirsch I and Weixel LJ (1988). Double-blind versus deceptive administration of a placebo. *Behavioral Neuroscience*, **102**, 319–323.

Luchelli PE, Cattaneo AD and Zattoni J (1978). Effect of capsule colour and order of administration on hypnotic treatments. *European Journal of Clinical Pharmacology*, **13**, 153–155.

Melander H, Ahlqvist-Rastad J, Meijer G and Beermann B (2003). Evidence b(i)ased medicine – selective reporting from studies sponsored by pharmaceutical industry: Review of studies in new drug applications. *British Medical Journal*, **326**, 1171–1173.

Moncrieff J, Wessely S and Hardy (2001). Antidepressants using active placebos (Cochrane Review). *Cochrane Database Systematic Review*, **2**, CD003012.

Moseley JB, O'Malley K, Petersen NJ, Menke TJ, Brody BA, Kuykendall DH, Hollingsworth JC, Ashton CM and Wray NP (2002). A controlled trial of arthroscopic surgery for osteoarthritis of the knee. *New England Journal of Medicine*, **347**, 81–88.

Nagao Y, Komia J, Kuroanagi K, Minaba Y and Susa A (1968). Effect of the color of analgesics on their therapeutic results. *Shikwa Gakuho*, **68**, 139–142.

Palace EM (1999). Response expectancy and sexual dysfunction. In: I Kirsch, ed. *How expectancies shape experience*, pp. 173–196. Washington, DC: American Psychological Association.

Pizzo PA, Robichaud KJ, Edwards BK, Schumaker C, Kramer BS and Johnson A (1983). Oral antibiotic prophylaxis in patients with cancer: a double-blind randomized placebo-controlled trial. *Journal of Pediatrics*, **102**, 125–133.

Pogge R (1963). The toxic placebo. *Medical Times*, **91**, 773–778.

Price DD and Barrell JJ (1999). Expectation and desire in pain and pain reduction. In: I Kirsch, ed. *How expectancies shape experience*, pp. 145–172. Washington, DC: American Psychological Association.

Rabkin JG, Markowitz JS, Stewart JW, McGrath PJ, Harrison W, Quitkin FM and Klein DF (1986). How blind is blind? Assessment of patient and doctor medication guesses in a placebo-controlled trial of imipramine and phenelzine. *Psychiatry Research*, **19**, 75–86.

Rickels K, Baumm C and Fales K (1964). Evaluation of placebo responses in psychiatric outpatients under two experimental conditions. In: PB Bradley, F Flugel and PH Hoch, eds. *Nero-psychopharmacology*, pp. 80–84. Amsterdam: Elsevier.

Rickels K, Hesbacher PT, Weise CC, Gray B and Feldman HS (1970). Pills and improvement: A study of placebo response in psychoneurotic outpatients. *Psychopharmacologia*, **16**, 318–328.

Schoenberger NE (1999). Expectancy and fear. In: I Kirsch, ed. *How expectancies shape experience*, pp. 125–144. Washington, DC: American Psychological Association.

Sodergren SC and Hyland ME (1999). Expectancy and asthma. In: I Kirsch, ed. *How expectancies shape experience*, pp. 197–212. Washington, DC: American Psychological Association.

Stewart-Williams S and Podd J (in press). The placebo effect: Dissolving the expectancy versus conditioning debate. *Psychological Bulletin*.

Traut EF and Passarelli EW (1957). Placebos in the treatment of rheumatoid arthritis and other rheumatic conditions. *Annals of the Rheumatic Diseases*, **16**, 18–22.

Watts RI, Freeman TB, Hauser RA, *et al.* (2001). A double-blind, randomized, controlled, multicenter clinical trial of the safety and efficacy of stereotaxic intrastriatal implantation of fetal porcine ventral mesencephalic tissue (Neurocelltum-PD) vs imitation surgery in patients with Parkinson's disease (PD). *Parkinsonism and Related Disorders*, **7**, S87.

Wolf S (1950). Effects of suggestion and conditioning on the action of chemical agents in human subjects – the pharmacology of placebos. *Journal of Clinical Investigation*, **29**, 100–109.

Chapter 5

Volition and psychosocial factors in illness behaviour

Robert Ferrari, Oliver Kwan, and Jon Friel

Introduction

Physicians (both psychiatrists and non-psychiatrists), psychologists, and other health-care practitioners have for decades been concerned with illness behaviour and the thought processing that underlies illness behaviour. One of the earliest environments in which clinicians found the need to describe and bring attention to these phenomena is in the medicolegal setting of injury, where symptoms and illness are evaluated within a compensation system. In this chapter, we review the historical examples from which clinicians have launched their quest to understand volition in illness behaviour; then we will use the clinical example of chronic whiplash syndrome to begin to formulate a construct of the interaction between individual, social systems, matters of gain, and thought processing in illness behaviour. We will conclude by examining the volitional aspects of illness behaviour.

Historical perspective

Illness behaviour was conceived by Parson (1964), adopted by Mechanic (Mechanic, 1960; Mechanic and Volkart, 1961) and subsequently expanded by Pilowsky (1997). These authors opined that symptoms manifest themselves in cultural substrata and are influenced by psychosocial factors. Illness has a personal meaning, and it seems intuitively correct that the personal meaning is sometimes thoughtfully examined by the patient, and thus presented to the health practitioner in a package that includes this evaluation.

Sir John Collie (1917) was among the first to make this observation. In one injured worker he noted the evaluation by the individual of the importance and relevance of their injury to the societal construct of workers' injury compensation:

> In short, the essential quality of a thing is its worth to the individual, and its value to him is its power to serve his private ends. On one occasion, when examining a working-man for an injury to his thumb, he observed me examining the terminal

phalanx of one of his fingers, which had been partially removed, obviously as the result of a former accident. 'That,' said he, 'is of no importance; it was done at home'!

The neurologist Kennedy (1930) then noted that motor vehicle collision or train collision victims held the strictest belief of being physically damaged, and seldom attributed any of their symptoms to any psychological factors, even when no physical injury was apparent. If the patient did acknowledge psychological disorder, they insisted that it was only secondary to the experience of chronic pain.

Denker (1939) also recognized the individual factors may together be instrumental in adoption of the sick role:

> . . . whatever his personal and family histories have been, any individual may find himself in a situation that tends to become progressively more unbearable and so predisposes to psychoneurotic conduct. A man working at tasks beyond his intellectual or physical capacity, or his emotional endurance, and harassed by obligations to carry on exhausting work without being able, from whatever ultimate maladjustments, to derive satisfaction from his work, this man is becoming predisposed toward a neurosis. Bare failure is intolerable; but failure camouflaged and compensated for by an illness that brings attention, sympathy, rest, and often an indemnity or wages without work is far from intolerable.

Rosenbaum (1982) similarly assimilated these observations and combined them with concepts of socially-acceptable criteria for sick role (see later) and secondary gain:

> 'Whiplash injury' is in style and begins with an actual physical disability. The patient does not produce the initial symptoms by psychological means, but instead captures the physical symptoms for psychological purposes. Today the patient does not simulate an illness; he has an illness, and he may hold on to this illness for secondary gains even after psychotherapy has helped with the presenting emotional symptoms.

Symptoms, illness behaviour, and the sick role

Symptoms

Symptoms are subject discomfort communicated to the observer(s). They are often ambiguous, and their interpretation involves a number of cognitive processes, which are subject to both psychological and social influences (Pennebaker, 1982; Cioffi, 1991). The experience of a bodily symptom initiates an active memory search in order to generate comparisons between the current stimulus and knowledge contained in the person's past experience and illness constructs (Leventhal et al., 1997). The outcome of this comparison process influences judgements about health status. Contextual and situational cues may also modify symptom interpretation by the provision of specific local information (e.g. other people with similar symptoms). This may also occur through culturally-determined illness schemas that cause selective attention to specific aspects of the symptom experience (Cioffi, 1991).

Causal attributions about symptoms are common and often reflect an interpretative process. The social environment may engender particular health concerns that bias both attention to bodily stimuli and choice of attribution (Barsky *et al.*, 2001). These factors, along with subsequent behavioural responses, are mediated by the interaction with factors such as mood, coping repertoire, available choices, and both situation-specific and general goals.

The common initial response is to assume that the symptoms will be short-lived and can be attributed to specific situational factors, but there are important individual and cultural differences in this respect (Robbins and Kirmayer, 1991). In the case of neck pain or headache after a motor vehicle collision, for example, the expectation of chronic pain afterward is culturally dependent (Ferrari *et al.*, 2002, 2003) and it has even been demonstrated that no collision is required for the syndrome to develop (Castro *et al.*, 2001). The need for seeking a physician is at least partly modulated by social factors (Cote *et al.*, 2001). As such, it is reflective of Sir John Collie's observation (1917) that the significance of, and attention to, a symptom or set of symptoms may depend more on what they mean (or their value) to the individual than on the biological underpinnings of the symptom itself.

Illness behaviour

Illness behaviour involves the manner in which individuals monitor their bodies, define and interpret their symptoms, take remedial action, and utilize resources of help as well as the more formal health care system (Mechanic, 1960). As such, illness behaviour is governed not only by the environmental factors (cultural, social, etc.). Pilowsky (1997) distinguishes between normal and abnormal illness behaviour. The individual with abnormal illness behaviour continues engaging in 'unusual or discordant, atypical behaviour conveys the type of illness behaviour that is more likely to reflect a personality or socioculturally determined style rather than a pathological entity'.

The sick role

Illness behaviour is the behavioural manifestation of adoption of sick role. Parsons (1964) defines the sick role as (Pilowsky, 1997):

> . . . a 'partially and conditionally legitimated state' which an individual may be granted, provided that he . . . recognizes his obligation to cooperate with others for the purpose of 'getting well' as soon as possible. Furthermore, he is expected to make use of the services of those whom society regards as competent to diagnose and treat illness.

Although the sick role derives from illness itself (an undesirable experience) the sick role may be desirable because it may have many benefits for the individual. It does, for example, absolve the individual from fault for their failure to meet obligations (Pilowsky, 1978):

> ... the sick person's disability and incapacity is not regarded as something for which he can be held responsible and is therefore not considered his fault . . . .

and (Pilowsky, 1969):

> ... he is exempted from his normal obligations to varying degrees.

Under certain circumstances, as Ford (1983) explains, the sick role offers a psychologically attractive option:

> ... the sick role is more attractive when (1) it is more culturally acceptable; (2) the social support system is perceived to be inadequate; (3) the individual feels under psychological stress; (4) the sick role resolves personal and social problems; (5) the individual is less self-reliant; and (6) coping skills are decreased.
>
> It is suggested that the sick role can be used to solve certain problems in living but that society does not accept emotional disorders or difficulties in coping with life problems to be an acceptable entry into the sick role.

It should be noted that these 'advantages' always exist in one's environment and are awarded, in the form of respite, as part of the social contract.

What are the criteria for the sick role? Because of the social stigmatization that exists towards most psychological illnesses, as being 'at fault', Ferrari and Kwan have explained that the sick role is most readily granted when the criteria of 'no-fault' is met (Ferrari and Kwan, 2001). It is implicit, as these authors describe, that a disease potentially influences one's behaviour largely beyond one's control. In such instance, the sick role, is granted.

If one has knee inflammation, one has knee pain. It is not under one's control and not one's fault. Ferrari and Kwan (2001) explain, however, that in society in general, many of the health-care gatekeepers, and often patients themselves, view psychological illness or disability as partially at least one's fault; their weaknesses, or their moral fortitude, are often called into question.

In most cases, one requires a no-fault entry into the sick role, and the appearance of organic illness (a disease) is certainly one of the most readily available forms. It is likely for this reason that the debate rages over fibromyalgia, chronic fatigue syndrome, late whiplash syndrome, etc., as disease versus non-disease, organic versus non-organic. If society would as readily grant the sick role to a patient with psychological illness with no stigmatization, then fibromyalgia patients would not have to constantly fight to legitimize their illness as organic disease. In the case of depression, society simply does not readily accept it as a disease, for the individual's own behaviour or lack of moral fortitude is held as his fault.

Even though one agrees that psychological suffering is still genuine suffering, labelling illness such as fibromyalgia as non-organic, psychological, etc. has the immediate effect of delegitimizing them as a no-fault entry into the sick role. And this bias is evident in both physicians and insurance offices. Even with the exact same label, with the same symptoms, and the same severity of symptoms, when the origin of the symptoms is considered to be emotional, disability is far less likely to be granted by the parties involved (Ferrari and Kwan, 1999).

So the sick role has this implicit admission requirement: present with something that appears to have a no-fault basis, usually looking like a disease (Ferrari and Kwan, 2001). One is obligated to minimize reporting of psychological symptoms or disturbances and maximize the reporting of physical symptoms such as pain, numbness, etc. that are seen in many diseases. If the patients admits to psychological disturbance, it is attributed as secondary to the pain, just as a patient with rheumatoid arthritis can develop depression secondary to chronic pain. Society accepts that the pain in rheumatoid arthritis is something beyond one's control, and so it is also beyond one's control if depression follows. It is probably beyond one's control in many other settings if depression occurs, but if a 'disease' is not there, society does not hold this view.

To enjoy the respite accorded to the sick role, one must be fully motivated to become well. Once the individual shows any motivations not to get well, then the contract is broken. For the individual to continue to behave as if he still has an illness and to demand consideration from his environment, the sick role is now being adopted. In its most extreme form, society labels the lack of motivation to get well (or motivation to remain ill) as malingering. In malingering, one consciously plots out and carries out one's conscious motivations, and is obviously in control of doing so. Is there another way to carry out one's motivations to maintain the sick role? There may be other ways indeed, and yet it seems odd that anyone would wish to be genuinely ill. It is understandable why the malingerer chooses to appear ill, because really they do not lose or suffer as a result of doing so.

Secondary gain and the economy of gain

The current meaning of secondary gain has, over time, become largely a legal concept; stemming from the social construct of the sick role. The general view of most people is that being ill is not desirable, and although there are gains to being ill (in this instance, secondary gains), there clearly are losses. This notion is incomplete. It is not uncommon for people to be suffering psychologically before they are known to be sick; they may hide their symptoms, perhaps even at times from themselves. They may have suffered many stressors, many miseries, many disappointments, and yet have to continue to cope with these losses and burdens, because society will not grant them any freedom to do otherwise (you need the sick role for freedom from burdens). Why then suffer with all those things and not be given the sick role when one can suffer with all those things (just change the presentation of symptoms from that of apparently psychological origin to that apparently of disease origin) and get the sick role?

To pursue secondary gain, the sequence may be as follows:

1 The sick role has criteria, those criteria are well known and are presumably over-learned in our society.

2 The secondary gains are available to those with the sick role, and are also presumably over-learned.

3 The sick role is available to those with no-fault entry (a no-fault illness).

4 The no-fault entry is thus available to those presenting with specified types of symptoms and syndromes.

5 One presents with those symptoms which may lead to a no-fault diagnosis (and minimize any symptom that might lead to an at-fault diagnosis).

6 Maintain that behaviour.

The question is, can this pursuit be achieved by means other than frank malingering – a largely conscious manoeuvre? From the dynamics of the model of consciousness states considered below, one appreciates that this is possible. But first, there is another phenomenon that must be considered before fully appreciating the mechanisms of adoption of the sick role – tertiary gain. The gatekeepers, for reasons other than professional and ethical ones, support patient's adoption of sick role (Kwan and Friel 2002) and, as such, play a significant role in the social phenomenon of disability syndrome.

Thought processing and illness behaviour

(Adapted with permission from Ferrari R (1999). *The whiplash encyclopedia. The facts and myths of whiplash*. Gaithersburg, Maryland: Aspen Publishers, Inc., pp. 484–497. © Aspen Publishers, Inc.)

Models of states of consciousness have been considered from a variety of perspectives. It is beyond the scope of this chapter to deal with each of these, or to fully address the sometimes confusing terminology in this broad body of literature. We will present a model based on Frenclian and current cognitive models.

Conscious state

The conscious state is equivalent to awareness and thus appears to be the state where thought processing is most amenable to control. Volition is synonymous with a capacity to control, or as otherwise stated a matter of free will. Control or volition does not necessarily require, however, conscious awareness of everything we are doing. It merely entails the availability of choices or alternatives. As long as we are aware of alternatives (or it is judged that we have the capacity to be aware of alternatives), then we have volition (Jang and Coles, 1995).

Unconscious state

The unconscious state has the special property of being entirely outside of our awareness and a collection of thoughts beyond our control, at least while in that state. According to the Freudian model, a model currently used in the courts, the unconscious thoughts are deep within our psyche and not readily accessible. It refers to those thoughts and thought processes that are incapable of being brought to awareness because of the operation of a counterforce. Such thoughts are kept, for example, in the unconscious state by psychic defences: they are repressed, at least for a time. Were they not repressed, and suddenly released, psychotic behaviour would probably ensue. They are potentially expressed over time through the development of a neurosis. The neurosis evolves when the unconscious thoughts result in excessive intrapsychic disturbance (i.e. anxiety and 'tension') that threatens to undermine the integrity of personality and ego functioning. This intrapsychic tension can be reduced by forming certain symptoms (so-called neurotic symptoms) and make it possible to preserve the greater part of one's integration. The preservation of integrity is termed primary gain, which lies in the mastery of otherwise overwhelming tension or anxiety; albeit at the cost of reduction of function and psychological effectiveness. Further, the development of a neurosis has the primary gain that the unconscious thoughts can be released in a non-psychotic manifestation, which is more gradual (often over months to years), and which is now amenable to eventual insight and adjustment. Otherwise, given their nature, unconscious thought processes are not generally accessible, except through psychoanalysis which may include dream analysis, hypnosis, etc.

If one cannot access one's unconscious thoughts, or control the events of primary gain, the neurosis must be, at least in large part, non-volitional. The courts have for years been using these two states (conscious and unconscious) as within a narrow version of the Freudian model, with thought processing believed to either exist in the conscious (fully aware) state or not. This is certainly an insufficient approximation of states of consciousness given present knowledge on the subject. Indeed, when Freud introduced the concept of the unconscious, it was not in terms of such a dichotomy (two-state model) (Civin and Lombardi, 1990). A third state – the preconscious – was considered an essential state, the function of which was to some extent intermediary.

Preconscious state

Freud first conceived the preconscious as merely a passageway from the unconscious to the conscious. Today, cognitive and experimental psychologists view the preconscious state in a more complex and yet practicable way. Thus, if the first step is abandoning the two-state model of conscious/unconscious, and recognizing the preconscious state, the second is viewing the preconscious state as evidenced by experimental psychology. Currently, the preconscious state of thought processing is characterized by unattended (unaware or unnoticed) information processing, that is the initial immediate analysis of one's environment (both external and internal). The thought processing is unattended (unaware) until its output has a mental representation (propositional or non-propositional), of which we are immediately aware (the thoughts are now attended) (Tzelgov, 1997). One can still retain some remnant of the aforementioned Freudian model by recognizing the unconscious state as the unnoticeable (unaware), that is repressed, and that cannot be brought to immediate awareness; while the preconscious state instead contains all that we know that is *not* repressed, and that can potentially be brought into consciousness without special effort (i.e. not requiring psychoanalysis, hypnosis, etc. to be brought to awareness) (Civin and Lombardi, 1990).

Velmans (1991), Kihlstrom (1987; 1993), and Dorpat (1983) have discussed how preconscious information processing may operate. In one aspect of this processing, information may be processed by focusing or not focusing attention on that information, the act of which may then bring a propositional representation to awareness (conscious). In denial, the preconscious information processing shifts attention away from, for example, disturbing stimuli emanating either from oneself or form the environment, to focus instead on less disturbing stimuli. This shifting of focus may occur at the preconscious level and may further allow thoughts that are disturbing to be repressed and placed in the unconscious state, psychic defences maintaining them where they are unnoticeable and no longer accessible. What determines how information processing leads to attention or not is, among many things, set by our prior experiences, our value system, our goals, our capacity to give sufficient attention to the information at a given time, and the overall significance or relevance to us personally of the information received or being processed (Velmans, 1991).

A pertinent stimulus, outside the focus of attention, can attract attention. If we could not determine the significance of stimuli outside the focus of attention, it would be difficult to know when we need to switch attention to them. We must have knowledge of the output of our information processing even though it takes place at a preconscious level. Learning allows for this process; state dependent learning notwithstanding. Thereby a preliminary analysis for meaning can take place outside of the focus of attention, without reportable consciousness (Velmans, 1991).

The preconscious information processing is thus monitored for propositional representations, that are then compared to our informational constraints, and attentional capacity, which in turn determine further how that information should be processed (that is one way we exert control, not so much over the information processing, but the evaluation of the output, and further processing of that output). Thus, automatic information processing itself is not within awareness, but the propositional representations are monitored and within awareness. This is the efficiency of the processing system, to allow for an apparent automaticity, the output of which can be monitored and thereby allows for input of control or constraints for further processing.

It seems clear that appreciating preconscious information processing is important in understanding certain aspects of illness behaviour. For, in the main, illness behaviour includes receiving and processing information both from within (perceiving a symptoms as painful, for example) and from without (information from one's culture including the health-care and social institutions, and the response of others to one's symptoms). Some aspect of processing of this information is probably preconscious. This model and its dynamics are depicted in Fig. 5.1. In the following sections, we discuss the extent to which this information processing is automatic, as that addresses the issue of volition in illness behaviour.

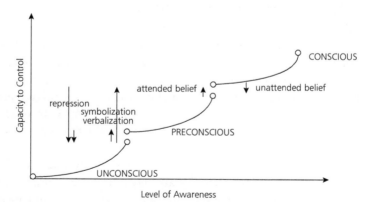

Fig. 5.1 States of consciousness – a quantized, discontinuous spectrum. (Adapted with permission from R Ferrari (1999). *The whiplash encyclopedia. The facts and myths of whiplash*. Gaithersburg, Maryland, Aspen Publishers, Inc., p. 489. ©Aspen Publishers, Inc.)

In the model, the trilogy of consciousness states are represented in this context as a spectrum of awareness and capacity to change by free will. The spectrum is discontinuous. That is, internal and external cues engage cerebral processes that gradually (the curved slope) build in intensity and distribution, until a threshold is reached, upon which the thought enters a different level of consciousness. This change in level of consciousness is instantaneous and renders a different capacity for the thought. This instantaneous and quantum level change thus reflects an infinite slope, hence the representation as a quantum level change and the discontinuity.

The change in quantum level is achieved by energy input, for example via symbolization in the case of changing from unconscious to preconscious or conscious. Equally, attending or unattending beliefs in response to internal or environmental cues (focusing or distracting attention, respectively) will precipitate a quantum level change.

The quantum level change from preconscious to conscious seems to be most readily achieved. This allows for one to have relatively automatic behaviour (unattended beliefs) so that daily events can be carried out based on previous learning, without demanding excessive energies or attention to those activities. When an environmental cue appears, however, it is necessary that those automatic behaviours be rapidly available to possibly adjust for the propositional representation output of preconscious processing (the belief becomes attended), so that a useful or desired change in behaviour can be effected. The attended belief, once the propositional representation is further processed and dealt with, can then become unattended once again.

Enacting of motivations of automaticity

Motivations are a form of readiness, and are goal-oriented (Pribram, 1995). Motivation means that there is a preparedness for action, merely waiting for the opportunity. Motivations reach into the individual's environment (Pribram, 1995). A motivation leads one to have an ever-present readiness to identify and further process environmental information that, taken together, suggest enactment of the motivation is possible. Clearly, in order for motivations to be enacted, they must lie within the realm of the preconscious and conscious, not the unconscious.

Automaticity may have a usefulness in enacting our motivations for desired goals in daily life. The preconscious state may thus be very important for processing of information within this more automatic realm. Automaticity is, however, vastly misunderstood for it is often held as synonymous with not requiring conscious input (Fleminger, 1992). If one imagines that adoption of the sick role, initially at least, involves the access to over-learned knowledge, a preconscious processing of gains versus losses, of attention to one's pain rather than to one's recovery, one wonders if it could remain as such, and be beyond one's awareness. In remaining at a preconscious level of processing, would the individual be aware of this behaviour? As we discussed above, for goal-oriented behaviour, it is more than likely they would.

The availability of secondary gain, as a part of the social construct of the sick role, is learned at an early age in most societies. This knowledge is held and integrated in our knowledge system though not always attended to. In this sense, such knowledge is said to be in our preconscious state and theoretically remains in all of us. The weighing of secondary gains and losses from illness may be a preconscious process. Most of us are not aware of going through the process of weighing the gains versus the losses as we begin to recover from our acute injury or illness. Yet, most of us, if we were asked now to make a list of secondary gains and losses from having chronic back pain could do so. We could then explain why we would prefer to be healthy, and why we would be motivated to become healthy. The knowledge is within us, and we are aware of the alternatives. Yet, we are not consciously aware of going through this after every acute back pain episode. To some extent, whomever granted us the sick role following acute injury is prepared to ensure access to secondary gains. Secondary gain is always there under such circumstances. How do we make that initial balance of gains and losses without being aware of it? It is likely that we do make such choices, but, at least initially, our own experience suggests that we do not initially process such information at a conscious level. We may later if we have a goal to reach and maintain.

The control of goal-oriented behaviour

Is the adoption of the sick role, as a social behaviour, a choice under one's control, or can it happen automatically, and be truly beyond one's control? For many years, just as there has been a perceived dichotomy of conscious–unconscious thought processes, there has been the misperception that these processes are either automatic or controlled.

The axiomatic definition of automaticity has long been that the thought process be unintentional, involuntary (lack of control), autonomous, and occurring outside awareness. In fact, most cognitive psychologists argue that the term automaticity should be abandoned in favour of the 'horsemen' of automaticity: unintentional, involuntary (lack of control), autonomy, and unaware. Behaviours may have some of the horsemen at work and not others.

Most social behaviour, therefore, often does not have all four of these horsemen at work. It is clear that most social and cognitive behaviours are complex and do not represent all-or-none phenomena, even though they may seem automatic (have some of the horsemen active) in some aspects (Bargh, 1989, 1992). To the extent that complex mental processes can become unmonitored or unaware through practice, the scope of preconscious processing may be expandable to some degree. Thus if one allows complex judgements to become routine, these may be performed even on subliminal stimuli being presented, especially if they are presented at the subjective rather than the objective threshold. Yet, this does not necessarily make them unintentional or uncontrollable. Bargh (1989) explains that although initial research on preconscious information processing has shown that social behaviours can be brought about without apparent effort, that same research indicates that experiment subjects needed specific instructions to make a judgement or form an impression. As such, they could not be unintentional. Bargh adds that other preconscious information processing experiments have shown measured behaviour to be unintentional, but dependent on effort of attention.

As a further example, consider driving. One is aware that one is driving, and one intends to drive. What makes this still seem 'automatic' while the qualities of unintentional and unawareness are lacking, are the other horsemen. There is autonomy of the action (once set in motion we do not have to be aware of how to keep it in motion), and there is a low level of attentive effort required (autonomy). Hence, as per the popular statement of an individual's elemental abilities: 'He can at least walk and chew gum at the same time.' This form of 'automaticity' (in one sense of the word) has been referred to by Bargh (1989, p. 24) as 'intended goal-dependent automaticity'. So if one is to consider automaticity, as still occurs in the courts and elsewhere, one must   further qualify which of the horsemen of automaticity is operative: unintentional, involuntary (lack of control), autonomy, and unaware.

Goal-dependent automaticity

The goal we have been considering here is adoption and then maintenance of the sick role. It seems paradoxical to have an 'intentional form of automaticity', but this simply refers to the fact that one may set a goal, and the process does not need to be controlled once it is started – it is autonomous. As Bargh (1989) points out, however, studies indicate that more attentional control and conscious decision making are needed when the situation has novel characteristics, or non-routine events arise. The fact that such processes immediately demand and attract conscious attention at these non-routine junctures indicates how closely controlled they are despite their otherwise autonomous nature. We suggest that over the lengthy process of adoption and maintenance of the sick role, such illness behaviour entails encountering many novel situations and non-routine events.

Illness brings events that entail losses that must be weighed each time they arrive, even though the loss may only be expected for a limited time. Alternatively there may be events that challenge the legitimacy of the sick role in some way, and those non-routine events must be dealt with to maintain the intended goal-oriented automaticity. The proximal stimulus of a consideration of gains that ultimately recognizes an economy favouring adoption of the sick role may very well be processed preconsciously. But control is necessary for the remainder of the behaviour to be maintained over time. Preconscious processing categorizes, evaluates, and imputes the meaning of social input – and this input is available for conscious and controlled judgement and behavioural decisions; however, those judgements and decisions are not mandatory and uncontrollable, given the proximal stimulus event alone (Bargh, 1989, p. 37).

It is true that while automaticity can be seen in some social behaviours in the experimental setting (Bargh *et al.*, 1996) in response to immediate stimuli, but this only occurs when the individual already associates a given situation with the behavioural representation being activated. The question is thus not how often such automatic behavioural events occur, but whether and how often they can be controlled or over-ridden by some conscious intention and purpose. We are all aware of the receipt of secondary gain as an expected consequence of illness, but the social behaviour of adoption of the sick role is not simply enacted by that awareness or even the existence of motivations for such behaviour alone. Fiske (1989) and Devine (1989) have suggested, for example, that the preconscious processing of prejudicial motivations, such as racial discrimination, require conscious input in order to be enacted. Although one may be able to affect a person's behaviour by making some motivations more salient than others, one cannot give the person a motivation that he or she does not already have and make him do something for which he or she has no motive base.

Conclusions

The sick role exists in most societies as a social contract between those who are not, granting relief from one's normal societal role during the illness. The contract may be broken when the ill individual is motivated not to 'get well'. Such motivations may arise for many reasons, but most generally from the economy of secondary gain. Certain individuals are at risk of having an economy that favours maintenance of the sick role because the secondary gains afforded by the sick role outweigh, in their personal value, the secondary losses from the illness.

The thought processing (cognition) underlying this behaviour can best be appreciated by considering the preconscious (processing to focus attention on thoughts related and cogent to the goal-oriented motivations) and conscious state (the thoughts that maintain and bind the process towards fulfilment of the goal-oriented motivations). Whereas much of the thought processing in illness behaviour may be preconscious and have some of the defining features of automaticity, such as autonomous (efficient), the overall behaviour, being goal-oriented towards adoption of the sick role, requires elements of non-automatic behaviour, such as intention, and therefore controllable behaviour.

The long-held field theory (Lewin, 1943) of social behaviour remains supported. The field theory holds that the individual must at some time (or many times) decide his motivations and determine the value of those motivations, and weigh the consequences of those motivations should they be enacted. Otherwise, the goal-oriented behaviour cannot be maintained. In order for preconscious processing to affect enactment of a motivation, it is necessary that relevant goal structures be activated. Thus, preconscious motivation to adopt the sick role would not be enough to achieve the illness behaviour which would ensure others grant the sick role. Even if one were to engage in the consideration of the economy of secondary gain at a preconscious level (outside one's awareness), the illness behaviour to adopt the sick role would not be chosen, unless the individual decides he wants the gains, and intends to pursue those gains (Bargh, 1996). Conscious awareness of motivations is necessary at some point in the evaluation process and in ultimately enacting the illness behaviour of adoption of the sick role. Further, it is the strength of motivations, and conscious appreciation of negative and positive consequences that determine the extent to which behaviours are enacted (Pribham, 1995).

Thus, most complex social behaviours have combinations of some of the features of automaticity, but not all features. This is what has lead to confusion about whether an act or behaviour is controllable or not. When an act is said to be outside of awareness, that does not mean on its own that it is fully automatic (all four horsemen involved), as it still may be intentional and motivated. Yet, many hold the misconception that lack of awareness of thought processes is equal to 'automatic' and assumed to thus be uncontrollable. Bargh (1996) point out that the view that there is a truly 'automatic' nature to social behaviours is falsely held because of the belief that automatic social behaviours are an all-or-none phenomenon. Complex social behaviours where one is laden with goal-oriented motivations (adoption of the sick role obviously being within this realm) necessarily require conscious control even though there are other horsemen of automaticity apparent. Preconscious processing does not remove control, but allows for the convenience and efficiency of some of the aspects of automaticity.

This interaction between the conscious and preconscious information processing to allow for the enactment of one's motivations to adopt the sick role may further explain the efficacy of cognitive therapy in chronic pain and other disability syndromes. There seems to be little doubt that belief systems, for example, influence the behaviour of chronic pain patients (Kilhstrom, 1987).These belief systems may be processed on both a preconscious (unattended) and conscious (attended) level. Cognitive therapy allows conscious efforts to alter the response to, and perhaps the very basis of, these belief systems through insight, further testimonial of the capacity of conscious thought processes to reach and thereby control the effect of preconscious information processing on enactment of one's motivations.

This same understanding allows for appropriate appreciation of the role that secondary gain plays in illness behaviours when it is 'not conscious'. We see that 'not conscious' does not equate with unconscious, nor does it necessarily equate with non-volitional or automatic either. The full appreciation of 'non-conscious' processes that are perhaps yet intentional and subject to volition arises only through an appreciation of the role of preconscious thought processing in illness behaviour – both its capabilities for aspects of automaticity, and its limitations in leading to motivation enactment and complex social behaviours. Indeed, understanding the interaction of automaticity, volition, and illness behaviour probably has numerous clinical, social, and legal applications.

References

Bargh JA (1989). Conditional automaticity: varieties of automatic influence in social perception and cognition. In: JS Uleman and JA Bargh, eds. *Unintended thought*, pp. 3–52. New York: Guilford Press.

Bargh JA (1992). The ecology of automaticity: toward establishing the conditions needed to produce automatic processing effects. *American Journal of Psychology*, **105**, 181–199.

Bargh JA, Chen M and Burrows L (1996). Automaticity of social behavior: direct effects of trait construct and stereotype activation on action. *Journal of Personality and Social Psychology*, **71**, 230–244.

Barsky AJ, Ahern DK, Bailey ED, Saintfort R, Liu EB and Peekna HM (2001). Hypochondriacal patients' appraisal of health and physical risks. *American Journal of Psychiatry*, **158**, 783–787.

Cioffi D (1991). Beyond attentional strategies: a cognitive–perceptual model of somatic interpretation. *Psychology Bulletin*, **109**, 25–41.

Civin M and Lombardi KL (1990). The preconscious and potential space. *Psychoanalytic Review*, **77**, 573–585.

Collie J (1917). *Malingering and feigned sickness*, 2nd ed, p. 258. London: Edward Arnold.

Cote P, Cassidy JD and Carroll L (2001). The treatment of neck and low back pain: who seeks care? Who goes where? *Medical Care*, **39**, 956–967.

Denker PG (1939). The prognosis of insured neurotics. *New York State Journal of Medicine*, **39**, 238–247.

Devine PG (1989). Stereotypes and prejudice: their automatic and controlled components. *Journal of Personality and Social Psychology*, **56**, 680–690.

Dorpat TL (1983). The cognitive arrest hypothesis of denial. *International Journal of Psychoanalysis*, **64**, 47–58.

Ferrari R (1999). *The whiplash encyclopedia. The facts and myths of whiplash*, pp. 484–497. Gaithersburg. Maryland: Aspen Publishers.

Ferrari R and Kwan O (1999). Fibromyalgia and physical and emotional trauma: how are they related? Comment on the article by Aaron *et al*. *Arthritis and Rheumatism*, **42**, 828–830.

Ferrari R and Kwan O (2001). The no-fault flavor of disability syndromes. *Medical Hypotheses*, **56**, 77–84.

Ferrari R and Lang CJ (2003). A cross-cultural comparison between Canada and Germany of symptom expectation for whiplash injury. *Journal of Spinal Disorders and Techniques*, **18**, 92–7.

Ferrari R, Obelieniene D, Russell AS, Darlington P, Gervais R and Green P (2002). Laypersons' expectation of the sequelae of whiplash injury. A cross-cultural comparative study between Canada and Lithuania. *Medical Science Monitor*, **11**, 728–734.

Ferrari R, Constantoyannis C and Papadakis N (2003). Laypersons' expectation of the sequelae of whiplash injury: A cross-cultural comparative study between Canada and Greece. *Medical Science Monitor*, **9**, 120–124.

Fiske ST (1989). Examining the role of intent: toward understanding its role in stereotyping and prejudice. In: JS Uleman and JA Bargh, eds. *Unintended thought*, pp. 253–83. New York: Guilford Press,.

Fleminger S (1992). Seeing is believing: the role of 'preconscious' perceptual processing in delusional misidentification. *British Journal of Psychiatry*, **160**, 293–303.

Ford CV (1983). *The somatizing disorders. Illness as a way of life*, p. 32. New York: Elsevier Biomedical.

Jang D and Coles EM (1995). The evolution and definition of the concept of 'automatism' in Canadian case law. *Medicine and the Law*, **14**, 221–238.

Kennedy F (1930). Neuroses following accident. *Bulletin of the New York Academy of Medicine*, **6**, 1–17.

Kilhstrom JF (1987). The cognitive unconscious. *Science*, **237**, 1445–1452.

Kihlstrom JF (1993). The psychological unconscious and the self. Experimental and theoretical studies of consciousness. *Ciba Foundation Symposium*, **174**, 147–167.

Leventhal H, Benyamini Y, Brownlee S, *et al*. (1997). Illness representations: theoretical foundations. In: KJ Petrie and J Weinman, eds. *Perceptions of health and illness*, pp. 19–46. Amsterdam: Harwood Academic Press.

Lewin K (1943). Defining the field at a given time. *Psychology Review*, **50**, 292–310.

Mechanic D (1960). The concept of illness behaviour. *Journal of Chronic Disease*, **15**, 189–194.

Mechanic D and Volkart EH (1961). Stress, illness behaviour, and the sick role. *American Sociological Review*, **26**, 51–58.

Parsons T (1964). *Social structure and personality*. London: Collier-MacMillan.

Pennebaker JW (1982). *The psychology of physical symptoms*. New York: Springer.

Pilowsky I (1969). Abnormal illness behaviour. *British Journal of Medical Psychology*, **42**, 347–351.

Pilowsky I (1978). A general classification of abnormal illness behaviours. *British Journal of Medical Psychology*, **51**, 131–137.

Pilowksy I (1997). *Abnormal illness behaviour*, pp. 39–41. New York: Wiley.

Pribram KH (1995). Brain models of mind. In: HR Kaplan and BJ Sadock, eds. *Comprehensive textbook of psychiatry*, 6th edn, p. 331. Baltimore: Williams and Wilkins.

Robbins JM and Kirmayer LJ (1991). Attributions of common somatic symptoms. *Psychological Medicine*, **21**, 1029–1045.

Rosenbaum JF (1982). Comments on 'chronic pain as a variant of depressive disease. The pan-prone disorder'. *Journal of Nervous and Mental Disease*, **170**, 412–414.

Tzelgov J (1997). Specifying the relations between automaticity and consciousness: a theoretical note. *Consciousness and Cognition*, **6**, 441–451.

Velmans M (1991). Is human information processing conscious? *Behavioral and Brain Sciences*, **14**, 651–726.

Chapter 6

Belief in rehabilitation, the hidden power for change

Derick T. Wade

Introduction

Suicide bombers, Kamikaze pilots, and martyrs all demonstrate that belief has more power to influence behaviour than almost any other single factor. Rehabilitation is, at its root, a process that aims to change behaviour of the patient and/or of others. Yet any suggestion that rehabilitation should using or, even more contentiously, changing patient beliefs should be an integral, legitimate part of the rehabilitation process is likely to raise eyebrows, if not hackles. This chapter discusses the importance of belief in rehabilitation from several points of view, drawing on evidence where it is available and known to the author. It suggests that the effectiveness of rehabilitation could be increased through harnessing the power of belief.

Beliefs held by a patient might have a powerful influence in several ways. The patient may have beliefs about the process of rehabilitation or specific therapies within rehabilitation that might influence, positively or otherwise, the effectiveness of the process and any treatments given. The patient may also have or develop beliefs about their own future and prognosis that may influence how much they undertake activities or attempt new activities. Patients may have, or develop, beliefs about the extent of their own influence on the process of change itself.

Beliefs held by others might also influence rehabilitation, either thorough affecting the patient or in other ways. The beliefs and expectations of family members may influence their own involvement, and may easily be transmitted to the patient. Similarly the expectations of professional staff and teams involved may have great influence. For example if the acute ward believes that people with multiple sclerosis (MS) cannot benefit from rehabilitation, then they will never refer anyone with MS for rehabilitation whatever recommendations are made. The beliefs and expectations of the members of the rehabilitation team may have a crucial effect. Lastly, the beliefs of purchasers of rehabilitation services will influence the nature and extent of any service bought.

What is belief?

The nature of belief is discussed in detail in Chapters 1–3. However, some discussion in the context of rehabilitation is needed. In terms of the World Health Organization ICF model (Wade and Halligan, 2004), beliefs can be considered as part of a patient's personal context; it is the set of expectations that they have concerning any particular situation. In this model, a belief may arise *de novo*, or be instilled by other people, or may arise from direct experience. Indeed, experience is presumably the most powerful determinant of expectations in most circumstances and determines the great majority of our actual expectations. The interpretation of experience may be judged faulty by others, but it is the individual's own interpretation that determines belief.

From the perspective of rehabilitation, the most important product of belief is the person's expectation of the future. Therefore beliefs are best reinterpreted as expectations, with belief simply being the (explanatory) intervening variable.

In terms of searching the medical literature, it is not easy! However the terms used in the searches for this chapter included:

- Self-efficacy – this can be construed as the belief in one's own ability to achieve and so representing the expectation (or otherwise) of being able to influence future states.
- Expectation – this is the consequence of belief; it is one way of defining belief.
- Belief.

Unfortunately searches were not very effective at identifying relevant literature, and one challenge for others is to develop a reasonable method for identifying relevant literature.

How might beliefs influence rehabilitation outcome?

Belief and expectation might alter the outcome of rehabilitation in many ways. The strong influence of the expectation of the observer – the observer's belief that a treatment will be effective – underlies the universal recommendation to use blinded observers in all evaluative research wherever possible. Ottenbacher and Jannell (1993) demonstrated that the effect size measured in studies of stroke rehabilitation interventions decreased the more unaware the observer was of the patient's treatment. Expectation biases the measurement of outcome by others.

Of course one could argue that the observers were simply dishonest, fabricating slightly better results. This seems unlikely. There was a consistent trend in the bias, with the bias being greatest when the observer was also the treating therapist and least when the observer did not know the patient's group, with independent but knowing observers giving intermediate bias. Moreover most people are intrinsically honest (or so I believe!). Finally, fabricated results are usually obvious and more extreme.

It is also well known that expectation may affect both how a patient reports their outcome and, more interestingly, their response to an intervention. In drug trials the so-called placebo response (which actually is the direct effect of patient belief) is a well-known and well-studied phenomenon (Harrington, 1999). In rehabilitation studies the placebo response is probably no less important when trying to design controlled investigations, but it is obviously much more difficult to blind patients to their treatment. In drug trials, the treatments (active and control) are identical, as far as the patient can tell. Achieving indistinguishable identity between rehabilitation interventions is probably impossible. Indeed, it should usually be impossible because patient participation in the treatment is an integral part of almost all rehabilitation therapies. Instead, in rehabilitation research, it is important to devise control interventions that are equally plausible to the patient; if this is not done the study may well simply be investigating the effect of differences in expectation rather than differences between the effectiveness of two specified interventions (Wade, 2005).

Although at least one meta-analysis suggests that the placebo effect is in fact small (Hróbjartsson and Gøtzsche, 2004), it does seem likely that expectation may influence measured outcome. For example in a study of a multidisciplinary intervention for Parkinson's disease which used a cross-over design, the group that were about to receive an intervention had a better emotional state that those who had completed their programme some 16 weeks earlier and did not expect further treatment (Wade *et al.*, 2003). One possible explanation is that the group expecting to receive their programme were more happy that those who did not expect any more.

Beliefs about outcome, and possibly the role of rehabilitation, certainly affect outcome. It is a commonplace observation that some patients simply 'give up' after an illness, believing that there is no hope. Research studies confirm the importance of belief, both about the prognosis and about the role of rehabilitation (Petrie *et al.*, 1996).

There is also some evidence concerning the power of belief in determining responsiveness to rehabilitation. The most striking was in a recent study where the patient's belief in the efficacy of therapy for back pain was noted to influence strongly the extent of response (Moffet *et al.*, 2005). Patients who believed strongly that physiotherapy would be most effective gained little from a cognitive behavioural treatment, whereas patients who preferred a cognitive approach and received it did very well.

The beliefs and expectations of others, both close friends and family, and other less close people such as work colleagues, and even professional health advisors, may also determine outcome. The most striking evidence of this comes from South Australia, (see Chapter 11) where a public health pro-gramme aimed at changing public expectations concerning acute back pain appeared to alter the likelihood of returning to work (Buchbinder *et al.*, 2001). This could simply have arisen from a direct effect of the education pro-gramme on the patient's expectations, but it is more likely that the general cul-tural attitudes and expectations of those around the patient also influenced decisions and outcomes.

A cynic could argue that all of these examples simply reflect 'biased observations' and that they do not demonstrate actual differences in 'real, true outcomes'. In the context of rehabilitation outcome, the 'real, true outcome' is usually the level of activities undertaken by a patient. This is usually established by asking the patient what they do, how well they do it, etc. Sometimes their activities are observed and quantified in some way. However, it is at least arguable that the patient's perceived activities (i.e. what they state that they do) are 'the truth'.

I would therefore conclude that beliefs alter the measured outcome of rehabilitation in several ways:

- Observations made by an external observer will be biased by their expectations of a particular intervention.
- The response of a patient to a specific intervention will be influenced by their expectations of that specific intervention.
- The response of patients to rehabilitation will be influenced by more general beliefs and expectations of others.

Determining beliefs and measuring their strength

Research into beliefs and expectations, and how they might alter behaviour and outcome (in the context of rehabilitation) depends entirely upon being able to identify specific beliefs and upon being able to quantify the strength of those beliefs. It is therefore important to consider how the expectations of a patient, and/or of their friends and family, and/or of their treating therapists might be determined and the strengths of those expectations quantified.

One simple way to establish the nature and strength of beliefs is to ask the appropriate question, such as 'How strongly do you believe (or expect) that this treatment will help you?', recording the answer using a visual analogue scale or numerical rating scale with two anchors such as 'Not at all' and 'very strongly'. Alternatively, one might ask the patient what factors they think might alter or affect their outcome, and then ask them to rate the strength of their belief in the same way. If there are several factors that someone thinks might alter outcome, they could also be asked to rank order them from 'most powerful effect' to 'least powerful effect'.

There are also established data collection tools that try to capture many different aspects of belief and expectation. For example there are generic and disease-specific 'locus of control' measures that establish the extent to which the patient believes that they have an influence over outcomes. There are many self-efficacy scales that measure the amount of influence that a patient believes they have over some aspect of their health. This chapter cannot review the many data collection tools available, and their strengths and weaknesses. Anyone interested in the topic should start by looking at other chapters in this book and at articles that study beliefs to discover how others have qualified and quantified belief.

However, when evaluating any data collection tool, and indeed when reading about the topic, it is important to remember that belief is only a construct deduced from behaviour and used to explain behaviour. Beliefs and expectations are not externally verifiable 'objects'. To that extent they are similar to most neurological impairments such as spasticity; any reader familiar with the great difficulty in agreeing a definition of spasticity, let alone agreeing how it is to be quantified, will appreciate the difficulty.

Does changing expectations alter outcome?

To the best of my knowledge no studies in rehabilitation have explicitly investigated this question. However, it is also difficult to undertake searches of the published literature. Nevertheless there are various arguments and strands of evidence that suggest that formal manipulation of beliefs could alter outcome.

An expectation of a change or specific outcome will usually (always?) be framed in terms of a specific state, some activities that can be undertaken, or roles that can be fulfilled. Once an expectation has been translated into a specific future state, it forms a goal, a state that the person is working towards. In so far as an expectation or belief relates to a specific outcome, then evidence concerning the influence of goals on behaviour becomes relevant. The evidence concerning goals and behaviour change is extensive (Locke and

Latham, 2002), and suggests that setting goals does change behaviour and that setting goals is more effective if:

- specific, not general goals are set
- challenging, not easy, goals are set
- long- and short-term goals are set
- feedback is given on progress towards goals
- the patient is committed, agreeing with goals
- the goals are appropriate to the situation.

Most of this evidence comes from outside health care, but there are now studies of goal setting in health care in general, and in neurological rehabilitation in particular, and the results are similar.

Therefore, it is probable that any intervention that changes a patient's expectation of (beliefs about) their outcome will influence that outcome. Indeed the process of goal setting itself could be considered one method of changing beliefs. The expert is assumed (by the patient) to know what can be achieved and is assumed to set achievable goals. In other words the patient is likely to adjust their expectations towards those suggested by others.

However, beliefs and expectations might also extend to the **process** of achieving goals, for example expecting change to occur 'naturally', or expecting 'therapy' to achieve goals without any effort on the part of the patient. One major expectation affecting outcome is probably the extent to which the patient feels that he or she has a part to play; the passive patient (often described as 'unmotivated') will generally do less well. There is some evidence that the setting a patient is in can influence their beliefs and apparent motivation (Maclean *et al.*, 2000). There is also some evidence that strategies that educate and involve patients in their own care may alter self-efficacy and it has been suggested that this may be the key intervening variable.

It is probable that the beliefs and expectations of the treating therapist or team will also affect the outcome of patients. In part, this can be a self-fulfilling prophecy or expectation. If a team believes that a patient will not (can not) benefit from their input, they will not assess or treat the patient and so, naturally, the patient will not benefit. However, a more common and subtle influence probably arises when setting goals; if the beliefs of therapists lead them to set challenging goals, the patient will do better. Moreover their attitude expressed during treatment sessions will undoubtedly affect the patient's attitude and expectations.

One may therefore conclude that changing beliefs (expectations) may and often will alter outcome:

- leading the patient to believe that they can achieve a more challenging goal will improve outcome (and the opposite is also true)
- leading the patient to believe that they personally can alter outcome, and need to be actively involved in rehabilitation will improve outcome (and the opposite is also true)
- leading the therapist or rehabilitation team to believe that their involvement will improve outcome will improve outcome (and the opposite is also true).

Beliefs about rehabilitation itself

The expectations generated by the word 'rehabilitation' may be a vital factor in determining many aspects of rehabilitation. Unfortunately, the word *rehabilitation* has no single agreed definition – it is frequently accompanied by the word 'physical', or the phrase 'physical medicine', both of which demote the importance of psychological factors such as beliefs; many people believe that it only applies to diseases that improve and recovery, excluding most neurological diseases other than stroke and head injury; many other people believe rehabilitation applies only to criminals, or only to people with psychiatric conditions, or only to people returning to sport, etc. – and few people take a broad view, using the word to encompass all aspects of helping people with illness to achieve their best within any limitations imposed by disease or other factors. Some reasonably frequent assumptions about (expectations of) rehabilitation are shown in Table 6.1.

This lack of understanding about rehabilitation, and lack of agreement about the aims of, processes involved in, and structures needed for rehabilitation may have quite severe consequences for the specialty and ultimately for patients. Perhaps the most important beliefs are those of the individuals and organizations responsible for funding rehabilitation. If they believe that rehabilitation is ineffective (despite good evidence to the contrary), or if they have a very circumscribed view of rehabilitation, or if they believe it should have a low priority then rehabilitation will be under-resourced (as it is now, in the UK at least). Politicians believe that science can cure cancer, and support almost any research and treatment; people believe that surgery and drugs are effective, and will pay for them, and there are many more examples.

Next, the beliefs of health-care workers not involved in rehabilitation are vitally important. Most patients are referred by staff working in other parts of the

Table 6.1 Some expectations of rehabilitation and their consequences

Expectation	Consequence
It is a process of restoration	The patient will return to normal Only patients who are expected to make some recovery 'naturally' should receive rehabilitation
Only applies to certain people	Only certain diagnoses referred Only people of certain ages referred No-one with illness referred (term only applies to prisoners, or building, or land etc)
Equivalent to therapy	Only referred if need a specific therapy, usually physiotherapy
Patient will be given treatment	Patient is passive and does not participate
Only applies to patient	Ignore family and/or carers Ignore environment and equipment
Only concentrates on motor function at basic level of personal activities ('physical')	Ignores emotional and cognitive problems Ignores work, leisure, social roles

health-care system. If they do not believe that rehabilitation has a role to play, they will not refer a patient who consequently cannot even be assessed to determine if they would benefit. Generally, it is also health-care professionals who are not involved in rehabilitation who will advise those who purchase health care.

Indeed, as I write this chapter, I have just seen a man who has been in an intensive care unit for 6 months and can move both arms reasonably (against gravity), breath, talk, and has full cognition though he still has a tracheostomy with some extra oxygen. His treating team apparently believed that he could not even leave an ITU in that state, let alone be rehabilitated home and so no referral had been made. By the time this chapter is printed, he will be rehabilitated home but their belief nearly prevented this outcome.

The beliefs of the patients and general public will also affect their expectations of rehabilitation, and their willingness to be involved or referred. A significant number of patients reject referral because they have a negative view of rehabilitation. Their beliefs will also influence politicians and those who fund rehabilitation. Although it may be paranoia on my part, I suspect that rehabilitation is not viewed very positively by most people both within and outside healthcare. Changing their beliefs might improve rehabilitation for patients.

Altering beliefs about rehabilitation

One way to improve the priority given to rehabilitation, and also to improve the use of rehabilitation services, is to alter the beliefs that people have about rehabilitation. This is extremely difficult.

Education and evidence might change beliefs, though probably only over generations. Explanations and definitions of rehabilitation have been given (Wade and de Jong, 2000). In summary, rehabilitation is:

◆ an active, educational, problem-solving **process**
◆ that is focused on a patient's **activities**, and
◆ that aims to maximize their **social participation**,
◆ while also minimizing the **stress on and distress of** both the patient and the family.

Moreover, the strength of evidence in favour of the effectiveness of rehabilitation is strong and well publicized, for example in relation to stroke, multiple sclerosis, and head injury but this approach has not led to much change.

As defined, rehabilitation has two objectives. The first is to increase the person's behavioural repertoire in their environment, maximizing what the person has the ability to do if they wish. The second is to ensure that they are aware of, and use, their abilities by ensuring that their goals are matched to their abilities (provided that the goals are socially acceptable). Another way of defining rehabilitation is as the process of helping the person to set achievable and socially acceptable goals, and then helping them to develop the behavioural repertoire needed to achieve those goals; it is a process of enablement, with the proviso that only achievable and acceptable goals should be enabled.

It is therefore possible to change the name attached to the process from *rehabilitation* to *enablement*. The word *enablement* has several advantages:

◆ It refers to a facilitatory process that involves the person concerned, and removes the assumption of passivity.
◆ It can refer to changes in:
  • the person's behavioural abilities
  • the person's environment (context)
  • the person's expectations or goals.
◆ It might persuade health services:
  • to be less prescriptive, and no longer to talk of compliance with, or acceptance of, rehabilitation
  • to be more patient-focused
  • to think more widely that *therapy*.
◆ It might help the patient realize that they are an active member of the team.
◆ It might also help the family to adopt a positive role.

Ultimately, it might change attitudes concerning the process from one where a health service has a duty to provide something to, or for, a patient to one where the health service has a responsibility to help the patient achieve something that is mutually agreed.

Conclusions

Currently, beliefs concerning rehabilitation, and the beliefs of patients within the rehabilitation process, are both probably reducing, rather than increasing, the benefits that could be achieved both for society and for individual patients. Within the rehabilitation process we should consider explicitly manipulating the patient's expectations to improve their outcome. We should also consider altering societal beliefs about rehabilitation. One way might be to use a new word, enablement.

References

Buchbinder R, Jolley D and Wyatt M (2001). Population based intervention to change back pain beliefs and disability: three part evaluation. *British Medical Journal*, **322**, 1516–1520.

Harrington A (1999). *The placebo effect*. Harvard University Press.

Hróbjartsson A and Gøtzsche PC (2004). Placebo interventions for all clinical conditions. *Cochrane Database Of Systematic Reviews*, **3**, CD003974.

Locke and Latham (2002). Building a practically useful theory of goal setting and task motivation. A 35-year odyssey. *American Psychologist*, **57**, 705–717.

Maclean-N, Pound-P, Wolfe-C and Rudd-A (2000). Qualitative analysis of stroke patients' motivation for rehabilitation. *British Medical Journal*, **321**, 1051–1054.

Moffett JAK, Jackson DA, Richmond S, Hanh S, Coulton S, Farrin A, Manca A and Torgerson DJ (2005). Randomised trial of a brief physiotherapy intervention compared with usual physiotherapy for neck pain patients: outcomes and patients' preference. *British Medical Journal*.

Ottenbacher KJ and Jannell S (1993). The results of clinical trials in stroke rehabilitation research. *Archives of Neurology*, **50**, 37–44.

Petrie KJ, Weinman J, Sharpe N and Buckley J (1996). Role of patients' view of their illness in predicting return to work and functioning after myocardial infarction: longitudinal study. *British Medical Journal*, **312**, 1191–1194.

Wade DT (2005). Randomised controlled trials in clinical rehabilitation. *Clinical Rehabilitation*, **19**(3), 233–236.

Wade DT and de Jong B (2000). Recent advances in rehabilitation. *British Medical Journal*, **320**, 1385–1358.

Wade DT and Halligan PW (2004). Do biomedical models of illness make for good healthcare systems? *British Medical Journal*, **329**, 1398–1401.

Wade DT, Gage H, Owen C, Trend P, Grossmith C and Kaye J (2003). Multidisciplinary rehabilitation for people with Parkinson's Disease: a randomised controlled trial. *Journal of Neurology, Neurosurgery, and Psychiatry*, **74**, 158–162.

Part 2

Clinical and occupational perspectives

Chapter 7

Public and medical beliefs about mental disorders and their treatment

Anthony F. Jorm and Kathleen M. Griffiths

The concept of mental health literacy

This chapter describes a programme of research on public beliefs about mental disorders which has been carried out using the concept of 'mental health literacy'. Mental health literacy has been defined as 'knowledge and beliefs about mental disorders which aid the recognition, management or prevention of these disorders' (Jorm et al., 1997a). Figure 7.1 shows a conceptual framework for mental health literacy. If a person experiences disabling psychological symptoms, or they have close contact with another person who has such problems, they will attempt to manage those symptoms. A person's symptom management activities will be influenced by their mental health literacy (arrow a). If successful, these symptom management activities may lead to a reduction in disabling symptoms and also a change in mental health literacy (arrow b).

In this framework, the person affected by the symptoms (either personally or through close contact) is seen as the primary agent in symptom management, with professional help being one of a range of strategies they might try. This view, which emphasizes the importance of public beliefs and actions, is a departure from previous thinking in the area. An interesting contrast is provided by the well-known Pathways to Care model of Goldberg and Huxley (1992), which has been very influential in guiding research on whether or not people with mental disorders get professional help. This model proposes that there are four filters that people with mental health problems pass through on the pathway from the community to specialist care. The first filter is illness behaviour which leads to help-seeking in primary care. If the person does not show illness behaviour they will not seek help from a GP. The second filter is the GP's ability to detect that the patient has a mental disorder. The third filter is the GP's decision to refer to specialist mental health services,

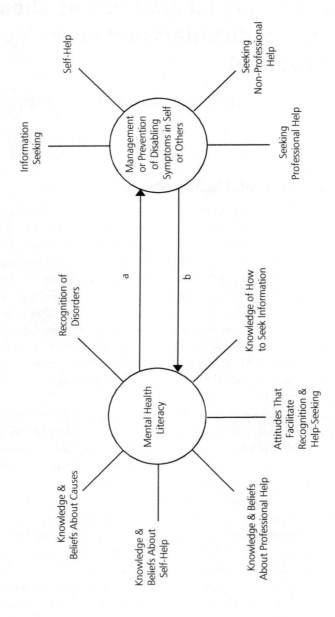

Fig. 7.1 A conceptual framework for mental health literacy.

and the fourth filter is the decision of specialist services on whether or not to admit the person to hospital. The viewpoint of the Pathways to Care model is very much that of the specialist psychiatrist working in a hospital who says 'How have my patients got to me?' It views the process as very much a doctor-driven one in which the only role of the person with the mental health problem is to show 'illness behaviour'. The person with the problem is viewed as largely passive. By contrast, the mental health literacy framework takes the perspective of the person who is affected by disabling symptoms and asks 'What can I do to feel better?', with seeking help from professionals being only one of a range of options. Whereas the Pathways to Care model emphasizes the need to improve the detection and management of mental disorders by GPs, the mental health literacy framework leads to a greater emphasis on increasing public knowledge and skills about mental health and empowering the person experiencing disabling symptoms.

The Australian national survey of mental health literacy

Because so little was known about public knowledge and beliefs, an Australian National Survey of Mental Health Literacy was carried out in 1995 (Jorm *et al.*, 1997a). This survey involved a nationally representative sample of over 2000 persons aged 18 or over. Respondents were presented with a vignette describing a person with depression or one with schizophrenia. No mention was made that the survey involved mental disorders. Respondents were asked what they thought was wrong with the person described in the vignette. While most recognized some sort of mental health problem, only a minority used the conventional psychiatric label. For the depression vignette, 39 per cent mentioned 'depression', 22 per cent 'stress', and 11 per cent a physical disorder. For the schizophrenia vignette, 27 per cent mentioned 'schizophrenia' or 'psychosis', but almost as many (26 per cent) mentioned 'depression'.

Respondents were next given a long list of actions the person in the vignette could take to help themselves. These included help from various professions and from family and friends, medications, psychological treatments, complementary therapies, and lifestyle changes. Respondents were asked to rate each of these actions as likely to be helpful, harmful, or neither for the person described in the vignette. The interventions that the public most often rated as likely to be helpful for the depression vignette were seeing a GP, a counsellor, help from close friends, becoming physically more active, getting out and about more, and courses on relaxation, stress management, meditation, or yoga. Two standard psychiatric treatments, antidepressant medication and ECT, were more likely to be rated as harmful than helpful. The results were similar for the schizophrenia vignette, with the interventions rated highest being seeing a counsellor, a GP, a psychiatrist, becoming physically more active, getting out and about more, courses or relaxation, stress management, meditation or yoga, and reading about people who have similar problems. Again, two standard treatments, antipsychotic medication and admission to the psychiatric ward of a hospital, were more often rated as harmful than helpful.

These results are not unique to Australia. Similar findings have emerged from surveys in Germany, Austria, the UK, Ireland, and the United States (Jorm *et al.*, 2000). In general, the public of many developed countries have very negative views about the benefits and risk of pharmacological treatments. However, they have much more positive views on psychological treatments, with many believing these are effective for psychotic disorders as well as for depression. Furthermore, complementary treatments are seen as effective more often than pharmacological ones.

Comparison of public beliefs with medical and other professional beliefs

These results suggested that there were some major discrepancies between public and professional beliefs. To see whether this was the case, postal surveys were carried out in Australia with national samples of GPs, psychiatrists, clinical psychologists, and mental health nurses, using the same questions that the public had responded to (Jorm *et al.*, 1997b, c; Caldwell and Jorm, 2000). As expected, the professionals consistently labelled the cases in the vignettes by the standard psychiatric labels. More interestingly, these surveys showed a remarkable consistency in the views of professionals about which interventions would be helpful for the persons described in the vignettes. For the depression vignette, at least two-thirds of each profession thought the person would be helped by a GP, a psychiatrist, a clinical psychologist, antidepressants, counselling, and cognitive-behaviour therapy. For the schizophrenia vignette, at least two-thirds of each profession thought the person would be helped by a GP, a psychiatrist, a clinical psychologist, antipsychotic medication, and admission to a psychiatric ward. While these views show some overlap with those of the public (e.g. the likely helpfulness of GPs and counselling), there are major discrepancies with other interventions, such as antidepressant and antipsychotic medication and admission to a psychiatric ward.

These discrepancies between public and medical beliefs have some important consequences. If people cannot recognize mental disorders and do not label them in the same way as medical practitioners, they may not receive any professional help or this help may be delayed. For example GPs are more likely to recognize depression in a patient who self-labels as depressed and specifically consults for psychological symptoms (Parslow and Jorm, 2002). It is also known that people are more likely to seek help if a relative or friend suggests it. Another consequence of the discrepancy between public and medical beliefs is that it places a limit on the implementation of evidence-based medicine. The idea behind evidence-based medicine is that patients will benefit if medical practitioners can be educated to provide care which is supported by scientific evidence as effective. However, this approach will only work if patients are willing to accept evidence-based care. There needs to be a concordance between the health practitioner and patient in how they think about the patient's illness and this requires that the public be given evidence-based information as well.

Belief systems about treatments for mental disorders

The contrast between public and professional beliefs about treatment suggests a continuum of mental health literacy ranging from expert knowledge at one extreme to complete ignorance at the other. However, even in the absence of specific knowledge of mental health, people may have general belief systems about health that they apply to mental health issues. The possibility that there are general belief systems emerged when factor analyses were carried out on ratings of the helpfulness of treatments (Jorm *et al.*, 1997d, 2000a). These analyses found three factors, labelled Medical, Psychological, and Lifestyle. Table 7.1 shows the treatment beliefs which loaded highly on each of these factors. A notable finding was that the same factors emerged whether the respondents were rating the depression vignette or the schizophrenia vignette. It is possible that the same factors might emerge for ratings of treatments for a physical disorder such as cancer, but data have not been collected to test this possibility. Obviously, these factors do not reflect specific knowledge about which interventions are effective, because each factor involves treatments that are supported by evidence as effective as well as ones that are not. Rather, it appears that if people lack specific knowledge, they then draw on general belief systems about health. For example if a person becomes depressed, but has little knowledge about depression, they may fall back on a general belief that the way to good health is to change lifestyle and that pills are unlikely to solve the problem.

Table 7.1 Treatment beliefs which loaded highly on each of the three factors

Factor	Treatment beliefs loading most highly
Medical	Antidepressants, pain relievers, antibiotics, sleeping pills, antipsychotics, tranquillisers, admission to psychiatric ward, ECT
Psychological	Counsellor, counselling, social worker, phone counselling, psychiatrist, psychologist, psychotherapy, hypnosis
Lifestyle	Help from family, help from friends, naturopath, vitamins, physical activity, getting out more, holiday, massage, new recreations

How can this finding of belief systems about treatment be reconciled with the concept of mental health literacy? People may start with general belief systems which form a scaffold on which specific knowledge is grafted. Rather than abandoning a general belief system, they might develop a more evidence-based version of it. For example a person with a strong medical belief system who develops depression and is treated successfully with antidepressants might still believe in medical interventions generally, but antidepressants become a more salient component of this belief system compared to other medical interventions (Jorm *et al.*, 2000a).

Belief and action

All of the research described above concerns responses to vignettes. Such responses are only of practical relevance if they predict what actions people take if they develop a mental health problem themselves or have to deal with it in someone close. To see if beliefs in response to a vignette predict action, a community survey was carried out which identified 422 persons with a high level of depressive and anxiety symptoms (Jorm *et al.*, 2000b). These people were asked their opinions about the helpfulness of treatments for a person in a depression vignette and then followed for 6 months to see if their beliefs predicted what actions they took to help themselves. The first column in Table 7.2 shows 34 interventions ranked for the percentage of respondents who rated each as likely to be helpful for the person in the vignette. The results are very similar to those of the Australian National Survey of Mental Health Literacy, except for the more positive response to antidepressants, which may reflect the fact that this was a sample of symptomatic persons who would be more likely to have personal experience of antidepressant medication. The second column in Table 7.2 shows the percentage of persons actually using each intervention to 'cope with stress, anxiety, depression or other emotional problems' over the 6 months of follow up. It is notable that some of the interventions that were rated highly for the vignette, were not actually used very often in practice, and *vice versa*. One reason for this discrepancy is that some interventions (e.g. consulting mental health professionals) are not easy to access for someone with mild symptoms. On the other hand, there are many self-help interventions which are readily available (e.g. alcohol) even though these might not be regarded as the most effective options. Perhaps the more important issue is whether those who rate a treatment as helpful for the person in the vignette are more likely to actually use this intervention themselves. For many interventions, this was found to be the case. For example those who believed that it would be helpful to have an alcoholic drink to

Table 7.2 Percentage of respondents (a) rating interventions as likely to be helpful for a depressed person in a vignette and (b) actually using the interventions to help themselves in the following 6 months

(a) Intervention (listed in rank order of helpfulness)	% Rating of intervention as helpful for vignette	(b) Intervention (listed in rank order of use)	% Actually using intervention themselves
Counselling	93	Occasional drink to relax	55
Counsellor	92	Pain relievers	55
Physical activity	91	Physical activity	50
Learn relaxation	90	Close friends	50
Close friends	88	Family	46
Cut commitments	84	Vitamins	43
Family	84	Time off work	40
Get out more	83	Get out more	35
New recreations	83	GP	35
GP	81	Cut commitments	33
Read about problem	80	Massage	30
Time off work	79	Read about problem	26
Massage	76	Special diet	22
Psychologist	70	Antidepressants	20
Telephone counselling	69	Chemist	18
Antidepressants	69	New recreations	16
Psychiatrist	67	Counselling	15
Vitamins	64	Sleeping pills	15
Social worker	64	Naturopath	14
Cut out alcohol	60	Counsellor	14
Clergy	58	Cut out alcohol	12
Psychotherapy	57	Antibiotics	11
Naturopath	54	Learn relaxation	6
Occasional drink to relax	46	Psychologist	5
Special diet	46	Clergy	5
Hypnosis	34	Tranquillisers	4
Chemist	32	Psychotherapy	4
Sleeping pills	25	Social worker	4

Table 7.2 (Continued)

(a) Intervention (listed in rank order of helpfulness)	% Rating of intervention as helpful for vignette	(b) Intervention (listed in rank order of use)	% Actually using intervention themselves
Pain relievers	17	Psychiatrist	3
Tranquillisers	11	Telephone counselling	3
Antipsychotics	11	Antipsychotics	1
Psychiatric ward	9	Hypnosis	1
Antibiotics	7	Psychiatric ward	1
ECT	4	ECT	0

Data adapted from Jorm et al. (2000b)

relax were twice as likely to use this intervention over the following 6 months as were those who believed antidepressants would be helpful. However, there were other interventions, such as seeing a GP, where responses to the vignette did not predict action, perhaps because there is little dissension from the general belief that seeing a GP will be helpful.

An 'overlapping waves of action' model

Another remarkable aspect of the findings in Table 7.2 is that self-help interventions predominate over professional ones. Of the 10 most frequently used interventions, all but one involves self-help. The most commonly used professional intervention is seeing a GP, which ranked ninth. It is paradoxical that many of these commonly used self-help interventions have received comparatively little research to evaluate their effectiveness, while some professional interventions have been extensively researched (e.g. psychotherapy) but are not so widely used in practice. We have argued above that there is a need for the mental health literacy of the public to be improved so that they are more willing to accept evidence-based treatments. However, there is also a need to develop an evidence base on these commonly used self-help treatments to better guide public action. This finding led us to do a systematic review of the evidence on self-help and complementary treatments for depression (Jorm et al., 2002) and to write a consumer guide to treatments to work for depression, which is described further below.

The findings about the frequent use of self-help also led us to do a further analysis of the actions that people take at different levels of severity of depression. There appears to be much that happens before a person consults a

GP or other health professional. To explore this issue we analysed data from a postal survey of over 6000 adults who reported on their current psychological distress and the actions they had taken in the previous 6 months to cope with depression (Jorm *et al.*, 2004). Figure 7.2 shows some examples of the results. As expected, professional treatments (such as seeing a GP, a counsellor or taking antidepressants) increase in frequency as symptoms become more severe. However, with some self-help treatments (such as engaging in enjoyable activities, physical exercise, and getting help from family and friends) there is an initial rise in use with increasing severity of symptoms followed by a drop in use at higher levels of severity. These findings led us to develop an 'overlapping waves of action' model of coping with psychological distress. According

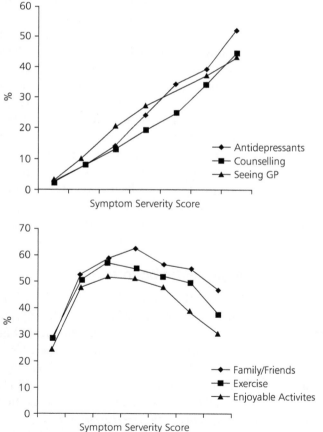

Fig. 7.2 Frequency of using some professional and self-help treatments for depression with increasing severity of symptoms.

Table 7.3 An 'overlapping waves of action' model for coping with psychological distress

Type of action	Level of distress where action peaks	Examples of this type of action
Increase existing self-help	Mild	Enjoyable activities, exercise, help from family and friends, music, eating chocolate
Adopt new self-help	Moderate	Vitamins, yoga, St John's wort, avoiding caffeine, fish oils
Seek professional help	Severe	See GP, counselling, antidepressants

to this model, individuals can take actions in any order or in any combination. However, in the population as a whole, certain waves of action can be seen, as summarized in Table 7.3. The first wave of action involves increasing use of self-help strategies that are readily available to the person and may already be in everyday use. This wave of action increases with mild distress, but then decreases as distress becomes more severe. The second wave of action involves self-help strategies that are not already in use and are adopted specifically to cope with distress. This wave peaks in moderate distress, then declines with more severe distress. The final wave of action involves professional help-seeking, which continues to increase as distress becomes more severe. It must be emphasized that these waves of action apply to a population and are not necessarily a sequence of actions for a given individual. Given that most of the action in the population is of the self-help variety, this model supports a greater emphasis on public mental health literacy, so that people with mental health problems can take more effective action to help themselves.

Interventions to change public beliefs

We have argued that mental health literacy is important for the better recognition of mental disorders, the adoption of effective self-help, and the acceptance of evidence-based professional help. The improvement of mental health literacy is therefore an important public health goal. There have been campaigns to improve mental health literacy in several countries, including the Defeat Depression and Changing Minds Campaigns in the UK (Paykel *et al.*, 1988; Crisp *et al.*, 2000), the Depression Awareness Recognition and Treatment (DART) Campaign and the National Depression Screening Day in the US (Regier *et al.*, 1988; Jacobs, 1995), the TIPS programme in Norway (Johannessen *et al.*, 2001), and the work of 'beyondblue' in Australia (Parslow and Jorm, 2002). Most of this work has involved broad community campaigns in which the dose of intervention received by an individual is typically small.

Also, the effectiveness of these campaigns is often uncertain. A complementary approach to broad community campaigns is to have more intensive interventions aimed at individuals. These are generally easier to evaluate using rigorous methodology. Here we describe a number of innovative approaches of this type.

Mental health first aid training

Many members of the public do first aid courses in order to learn how to handle medical emergencies. However, these courses typically ignore mental health issues, despite the high incidence of mental health problems in the community. To fill this gap, Kitchener and Jorm (2002a) have developed a Mental Health First Aid course dealing with mental health crisis situations and early assistance to people developing a mental disorder. The crisis situations covered are: suicidal thoughts, panic attack, exposure to a traumatic event, psychotic person threatening violence, and drug overdose. The course also teaches what assistance can be provided to people developing depression, anxiety disorder, psychosis, and substance misuse. The course involves applying the following steps to each of these mental health problems:

- Assess risk of suicide or harm
- Listen non-judgmentally
- Give reassurance and information
- Encourage the person to get appropriate professional help
- Encourage self-help strategies

An uncontrolled evaluation of Mental Health First Aid has been carried out based on questionnaires given before the course, at the end, and 6 months after (Kitchener and Jorm, 2002b). This evaluation showed that the course improved participants' ability to recognize a mental disorder in a vignette, changed beliefs about treatment so that they became more like those of health professionals, decreased stigma, increased confidence in providing help to others, and increased the actual amount of help provided to others.

This evaluation did not involve a control group. However, there are two randomized controlled trials underway in which Mental Health First Aid is compared to wait-list control groups. One of these trials involves employees in a government department and the other involves members of the public in a large rural area in Australia.

The Mental Health First Aid course is now widely available in Australia, where it is run mainly on a fee-for-service basis, and it has spread to the UK.

A consumer guide to treatments for depression

Many information and self-help books and brochures have been developed for mental health consumers. However, few are evidence-based and those which are tend to focus on a limited range of treatments. We therefore set about developing a comprehensive, evidence-based consumer guide to conventional and self-help treatments. Based on a systematic review of the literature, the resulting guide, *Help for depression: What Works (and What Doesn't)* (Jorm *et al.*, 2001) provides the public with evidence abut the effectiveness of 45 medical, psychological, and alternative treatments for depression. Details of the review methodology are available in Jorm *et al.* (2002).

The guide, which is written at year 8 level, describes each intervention, its hypothesized mechanism of action, the evidence for its effectiveness, dis-advantages (including side-effects), where it can be obtained, whether it is recommended, and key references. Each intervention is accompanied by a five-point visual rating scale that ranges from three smiley faces for a treatment for which there is good evidence of effectiveness to a straight face for ineffective interventions and a question mark for intervention that have not been subjected to scientific evaluation.

Jorm *et al.* (2003) conducted a randomized, controlled trial of the effect of the guide on 1094 people from the community who screened positive for elevated depressive symptoms. Participants were randomized to receive either the evidence-based guide or a five-page government brochure on depression (control brochure). The guide was rated by participants as more useful than the control brochure and those receiving the guide were more likely to report that they took action because of it (and, in particular, did something differently, tried self-help treatments, gave advice to someone). The *What Works* guide was also associated with greater improvement in knowledge about the effectiveness of some treat-ments. However, there was no difference in the effect of the guide and control brochures on depressive symptoms or disability ratings. There are a number of possible reasons why the depressive symptoms did not show greater improvement for the *What Works* intervention. First, it is possible that the control condition was actually of some benefit since the government brochure did include some evidence-based information. Other factors that may have contributed to an absence of effects for depressive symptoms include the high participant drop out rate, the possibility that participants did not read all the material, and a small effect size that might have been detectable with a larger trial.

Use of the internet to change public beliefs

A substantial percentage of the community now has access to the internet (Taylor, 2003; ABS, 2003). Increasingly, internet users are seeking health informa-tion online (Taylor, 2002). According to a Harris Poll, 80 per cent of online users have sought health information on the web (Taylor, 2002). Significantly, it has been reported that information about depression is the most common reason for accessing online information about a health condition. Moreover, 43 per cent of people report that they were seeking information about a mental disorder when they last accessed health information on the web (Taylor, 1999).

Clearly, the web offers an important opportunity to disseminate to the public, accurate up-to-date information on mental health conditions, and depression in particular. In fact, there are many thousands of web sites on depression. However, systematic studies have demonstrated that these web sites are typically of poor quality when compared to evidence-based guidelines (Griffiths and Christensen, 2000, 2002). To address this problem, we developed the evidence-based depression web site, BluePages (http://bluepages.anu.edu.au). Like the *What Works* consumer guide, BluePages contains evidence-based information about medical, psychological, and alternative treatments. It also includes information about symptoms and the experience of depression, information about sources of help and other key resources. It incorporates online anxiety and depression screening tests and norms and a state-of-the art search engine that allows focused search across more than 100 depression sites.

The ultimate test of the quality of a health website is whether it leads to improved health outcomes. To date, there are no published evaluations of the effect of any of the numerous psychoeducational depression web sites on attitudes, behaviours, or symptoms. Accordingly, we have recently conducted a randomized, controlled trial of BluePages to evaluate its effectiveness in reducing depressive symptoms, increasing depression literacy, and decreasing stigma. A large number of participants from the community who screened positive for elevated levels of depression symptoms were randomly assigned to receive one of three interventions: BluePages; MoodGYM, a website delivering cognitive behavioural therapy; or an Attention Control in which they were interviewed weekly on the telephone. The results of this study showed that BluePages increased understanding of depression treatments and also reduced depressive symptoms (Christensen *et al*, 2004). It is likely that with effective dissemination, an information intervention such as BluePages could have a major impact at the population level (Jorm *et al.*, 2003).

Conclusions

The theme of this chapter is the importance of beliefs in medicine. The programme of research described here illustrates this theme quite well. We have shown that the public tends to think differently from medical and other health professionals about treatments for mental disorders. These differences affect what actions people take, including their willingness to take evidence-based treatments. Even when the members of the public have no specific knowledge of mental health, they do not act in a vacuum. They have general belief systems about health which are called into play in the absence of specific knowledge. Given the limitation which public beliefs place on the implementation of evidence-based medicine, improving mental health literacy needs to be an important public health goal. There are a range of options for achieving this, including community-wide media campaigns, individual training courses, evidence-based consumer guides, and high quality information on the internet. Improving mental health literacy has the potential to decrease the prevalence of untreated disorders, to improve the uptake of optimal treatment and self-care.

References

Australian Bureau of Statistics (ABS) (2003). *Internet activity, Australia*. March Quarter, 2003 (8153.0). Canberra: Australian Bureau of Statistics.

Caldwell TM and Jorm AF (2000). Mental health nurses' beliefs about interventions for schizophrenia and depression: A comparison with psychiatrists and the public. *Australian and New Zealand Journal of Psychiatry*, **34**, 602–611.

Christensen H, Griffiths KM and Jorm AF (2004). Delivering interventions for depression by using the internet: randomised controlled trial. *British Medical Journal*, **328**, 265.

Crisp AH, Gelder MG, Rix S, Meltzer HI and Rowlands OJ (2000). Stigmatisation of people with mental illnesses. *British Journal of Psychiatry*, **177**, 4–7.

Goldberg D and Huxley P (1992). *Common mental disorders: A bio-social model*. London and New York: Routledge.

Griffiths KM and Christensen H (2000). Quality of Web based information on treatment of depression: cross sectional survey. *British Medical Journal*, **321**, 1511–1515.

Griffiths KM and Christensen H (2002). The quality of Australian depression Web sites. *Medical Journal of Australia*, **176**, S97–S104.

Jacobs DG (1995). National depression screening day: Educating the public, reaching those in need of treatment, and broadening professional understanding. *Harvard Review of Psychiatry*, **3**, 156–159.

Johannessen JO, McGlashan TH, Larsen TK, Horneland M, Joa I, Mardal S, Kvebaek R, Friis S, Melle I, Opjordsmoen S, Simonsen E, Ulrik H and Vaglum P (2001). Early detection strategies for untreated first-episode psychosis. *Schizophrenia Research*, **51**, 39–46.

Jorm AF, Angermeyer M and Katschnig H (2000). Public knowledge of and attitudes to mental disorders: A limiting factor in the optimal use of treatment services. In: G Andrews and AS Henderson, eds. *Unmet need in psychiatry*, pp. 399–413. Cambridge: Cambridge University Press.

Jorm AF, Christensen H, Griffiths KM, Korten AE and Rodgers B (2001). *Help for depression: what works (and what doesn't)*. Canberra: Centre for Mental Health Research.

Jorm AF, Christensen H, Griffiths KM and Rodgers B (2002). Effectiveness of complementary and self-help treatments for depression. *Medical Journal of Australia*, **176**, S84–S96.

Jorm AF, Christensen H, Medway J, Korten AE, Jacomb PA and Rodgers B (2000a). Public belief systems about the helpfulness of interventions for depression: Associations with history of depression and professional help-seeking. *Social Psychiatry and Psychiatric Epidemiology*, **35**, 211–219.

Jorm AF, Griffiths KM, Christensen H, Korten AE, Parslow RA and Rodgers B (2003). Providing information about the effectiveness of treatment options to depressed people in the community: A randomized controlled trial of effects on mental health literacy, help-seeking and symptoms. *Psychological Medicine*, **33**, 1071–1087.

Jorm AF, Griffiths KM, Christensen H, Parslow RA and Rodgers B (2004). Actions taken to cope with depression at different levels of severity: A community survey. *Psychological Medicine*, **34**, 293–299.

Jorm AF, Korten AE, Jacomb PA, Christensen H, Rodgers B and Pollitt P (1997a). 'Mental health literacy': a survey of the public's ability to recognise mental disorders and their beliefs about the effectiveness of treatment. *Medical Journal of Australia*, **166**, 182–186.

Jorm AF, Korten AE, Jacomb PA, Rodgers B and Pollitt P (1997c). Beliefs about the helpfulness of interventions for mental disorders: a comparison of general practitioners, psychiatrists and clinical psychologists. *Australian and New Zealand Journal of Psychiatry*, **31**, 844–851.

Jorm AF, Korten AE, Jacomb PA, Rodgers B, Pollitt P, Christensen H and Henderson S (1997b). Helpfulness of interventions for mental disorders: Beliefs of health professionals compared with the general public. *British Journal of Psychiatry*, **171**, 233–237.

Jorm AF, Korten AE, Rodgers B, Pollitt P, Jacomb PA, Christensen H and Jiao Z (1997d). Belief systems of the general public concerning the appropriate treatments for mental disorders. *Social Psychiatry and Psychiatric Epidemiology*, **32**, 468–473.

Jorm AF, Medway J, Christensen H, Korten AE, Jacomb PA and Rodgers B (2000b). Public beliefs about the helpfulness of interventions for depression: Effects on actions taken when experiencing anxiety and depression symptoms. *Australian and New Zealand Journal of Psychiatry*, **34**, 619–626.

Kitchener BA and Jorm AF (2002a). *Mental health first aid manual*. Canberra: Centre for Mental Health Research.

Kitchener BA and Jorm AF (2002b). Mental health first aid training for the public: evaluation of effects on knowledge, attitudes and helping behavior. *BMC Psychiatry*, **2**, 10.

Parslow RA and Jorm AF (2002). Improving Australians' depression literacy. *Medical Journal of Australia*, **177**, S117–S121.

Paykel ES, Hart D and Priest RG (1988). Changes in public attitudes to depression during the defeat depression campaign. *British Journal of Psychiatry*, **173**, 519–522.

Regier DA, Hirschfeld RMA, Goodwin FK, Burke JD, Lazar JB and Judd LL (1988). The NIMH depression awareness, recognition, and treatment program: Structure, aims, and scientific basis. *American Journal of Psychiatry*, **145**, 1351–1357.

Taylor H (1999). Explosive growth of 'cyberchondriacs'. *The Harris Poll*, 47. URL: http://www.harrisinteractive.com/harris_poll/index.asp?PID=117, last accessed 18 September, 2003.

Taylor H (2002). Cyberchondriacs update. *The Harris Poll*, 21. URL: http://www.harrisinteractive.com/harris_poll/index.asp?PID= 299, last accessed 18 September, 2003.

Taylor H (2003). Those with internet access to continue to grow but at a slower rate. *The Harris Poll*, 8. URL: http://www.harrisinteractive.com/harris_poll/index.asp?PID=356, last accessed 18 September, 2003.

Chapter 8

Beliefs and adherence to treatment: the challenge for research and clinical practice

Rob Horne

Introduction

Not all treatments work for everyone. People with the same disease do not respond to the same treatment in the same way. Variation in response between (and within) individuals is a key challenge for medical science, yet it has received relatively little attention compared to efforts to develop new and innovative treatments. This is understandable but inefficient. The search for new and better treatments should go hand in hand with efforts to maximize the benefits of existing treatments. In this chapter I will argue that we are failing to do this and suggest ways in which we might improve the situation through a better understanding of how patients perceive and think about treatments.

There are clear pharmacological and physiological reasons for individual variation in response to medication. However, this is not the whole story. As with most medical phenomena, psychological factors are also important. There is increasing recognition that beliefs influence response to treatment in at least two major ways. They have a direct effect on outcomes through the placebo and nocebo effects and they have an indirect effect by influencing behaviour: determining what the patient does with the treatment and whether they adhere to the prescriber's recommendations. Placebo effects are well recognized in medicine but poorly understood and this fascinating topic is dealt with in Chapter 4 of this volume. In this chapter, I will focus on the role of beliefs in determining treatment-related behaviours.

I will take pharmaceutical medicines as my main example. Over the last 50 years or so, the development of pharmaceuticals has revolutionized the treatment of common diseases. Their prescription is now one of the most common medical interventions, and, in many countries, the single biggest source of expenditure after healthcare staff. However, much of this medication is unused. Hippocrates observations that many patients do not adhere to physicians treatment recommendations was recently updated in a comprehensive review of adherence in long-term medical conditions compiled by the World Health Organization (2003).

Non-adherence to treatment: the scale of the problem

In affluent countries, most health resources are spent on the management of chronic diseases such as coronary heart disease, diabetes, and asthma. Here, good outcomes depend as much on self-management as on good medical care and, for most of these conditions, self-management hinges on the appropriate use of medicines. But it is thought that over a third of prescribed medicines are not taken as directed. Non-adherence is a concern for those providing, receiving. or funding healthcare because it not only entails a waste of resources but also a missed opportunity for therapeutic benefit. However, few effective interventions to facilitate adherence have been developed (Haynes *et al.*, 2004) and there is increasing interest in understanding the causes of nonadherence.

Understanding non-adherence: the importance of patients' beliefs

The non-adherent patient – a myth

Non-adherence is not significantly related to the type or severity of disease, with rates of between 25 and 30 per cent noted across 17 disease conditions (DiMatteo, 2004). Furthermore, providing clear information – although essential – is not enough to guarantee adherence (Weinman, 1990). Likewise, a research has failed to identify clear and consistent relations between adherence and sociodemographic variables, such as gender and age in adults. Adherence is positively correlated with income when medication has to be purchased directly by the patient (Piette *et al.*, 2004) but not with general socioeconomic status (DiMatteo, 2004).

There is little evidence that adherence behaviours can be explained in terms of trait personality characteristics. Even if stable associations existed between sociodemographic or trait characteristics, they would serve to identify certain 'at risk' groups to facilitate targeting of interventions but could do little to inform the type or content of interventions. This is not to say that sociodemographic or dispositional characteristics are irrelevant. Rather it would seem that associations with adherence may be indirect and best explained by the influence of sociodemographic and dispositional characterizes on other relevant parameters. For example correlations between adherence and educational status or race may simply be a reflection of income and ability to afford prescription costs. In summary then, the notion of a typical 'non-adherent patient' is something of a myth: most patients are non-adherent some of the time. Stable characteristics, such as the nature of the disease and treatment or sociodemographic variables, influence the adherence behaviour of some patients more than others. This has led to a greater emphasis on understanding the interaction of the individual with the disease and treatment, rather than identifying the characteristics of the 'non-adherent patient'.

The gap between knowing and doing: intentional and unintentional non-adherence

Non-adherence can be thought of as two related types of behaviour:

Unintentional – when patients intentions to take the medication as advised are thwarted by barriers that are essentially beyond their control, such as forgetful-ness, poor comprehension language barriers, or physical inability to manage the medication (e.g. difficulties opening containers or using administration devices).

Intentional – a conscious decision by the patient to take the medication in a way which differs from instructions, or not to take it all. This often takes the form of patients reducing the frequency of dosing or the number of medications down to a level that they (and not their doctor) feel is appropriate, or prema-ture discontinuation of therapy.

This simple model is useful because it helps us to begin to understand the type of interventions that are needed to help patients get the best from medicines and to understand why previous attempts have had only limited effects (Haynes *et al.*). Using medication appropriately is essentially dependent on two factors: *ability* and *motivation*. Unintentional non-adherence is essentially a problem of ability. A range of interventions have been developed to address this problem including issuing reminders, simplifying the regimen, or providing clear instructions. These are useful and help many patients. However, one reason why published interventions to promote adherence have met with relatively little success is that they tend to target patient ability and resources yet ignore motivation.

Several theoretical models have been developed to explain how people initiate and maintain actions to preserve or improve health status. These models share the common assumption that the motivation to engage in and maintain health-related behaviours arises from beliefs that influence the interpretation of information and experiences and guide behaviour (see Conner and Norman, 1996 for a review of social cognition models; and Horne and Weinman, 1998 for an overview of theoretical models applied to adherence).

The present chapter will describe a simple framework for conceptualizing the specific treatment beliefs that may be particularly salient to adherence and summarizes empirical evaluations of this framework in relation to medication adherence. It will then consider the role of treatment beliefs in the self-regulation of illness and outline the implications for future research and practice.

Beliefs about medicines

Given the importance of medicines in health care and the apparently widespread problem of non-adherence, surprisingly little attention has focused on how people perceive and make decisions about medicines. There are a few notable exceptions (see Horne, 1997 for a review). Several seminal studies had used qualitative methods to explore people's perceptions of medications (Arluke, 1980; Coulter, 1985; Gabe and Lipshitz Phillips, 1982; Morgan and Watkins, 1988). There were interesting similarities in people's ideas about medicines (e.g. that medicines are addictive and accumulate within the body to produce 'long-term' effects) that seemed to be common across locations and cultures (US, UK, and other European countries) and illness/treatment categories (Horne, 1997).

These studies led us to question whether the commonly-expressed beliefs about prescribed medicines could be summarized under simple core themes. We therefore began our investigation of medication beliefs by exploring the principal components underlying representations of prescribed medication. These analyses showed that, although patients' ideas about medicines are often complex and diverse, many of the beliefs relating to prescribed medication could be grouped under two categories: perceptions of *necessity* or personal need for the treatment, and *concerns* about negative effects (Horne et al., 1999).

Necessity beliefs

Studies across medical conditions show that people prescribed the same medication for the same condition, differ in their perceptions of personal need for it (Horne et al., 1999). Necessity beliefs are operationialized by statements such as 'My health depends on this medicine', 'These medicines protect me from becoming worse' and 'Without these medicines I would be very ill'. It is worth noting that perceived necessity is not a form of efficacy belief (a belief about whether the treatment will be effective). Although views about efficacy are likely to contribute to perceived need, the constructs are not synonymous. We might believe that a treatment will be effective but yet not perceive a personal *need* for it. Conversely, we might perceive a strong need for a treatment that we perceive to be only moderately effective, because we know that it is the only treatment that is available. We anticipate that *necessity* beliefs will be more closely related to adherence than beliefs about treatment efficacy.

Concerns about medication

There is a striking similarity in the type of concerns that patients report about prescription medicines. One obvious source of concern is the experience of unpleasant symptoms as medication 'side-effects' and the disruptive effects of medication on daily living; but this is not the whole picture. Many patients receiving regular medication who have not experienced adverse effects are still worried about possible problems in the future. These often arise from the commonly held belief that regular use can lead to dependence or that the medication will accumulate within the body and lead to harmful, long-term effects. These core concerns seem to be fairly generic and relevant across a range of disease states and cultures, and they are typically endorsed by over a third of study participants (Horne *et al.*, 2001c; Horne *et al.*, 2004; Horne and Weinman, 1999). Other concerns are specific to the particular class of medicine (Horne and Weinman, 2002). For example worries that corticosteroid inhalers prescribed for asthma will result in weight gain (Hand and Bradley, 1996) or that regular use of analgesic medication now will make it less effective in the future (Gill and Williams, 2001).

Beliefs about prescribed medication as barriers to adherence: balancing necessity beliefs and concerns

Studies involving patients from a wide range of illness groups, including: asthma (Horne and Weinman, 2002), renal disease (Horne *et al.*, 2001c), diabetes (Horne and Weinman, 1999), coronary heart disease (Horne and Weinman, 1999), hypertension (Ross *et al.*, 2004), HIV/Aids (Horne *et al.*, 2004), and haemophilia (Llewellyn *et al.*, 2003), have consistently found that low rates of adherence were related to doubts about personal need for medication and concerns about potential adverse effects.

The negative correlation between concerns and reported adherence suggests that patients may respond to fears about potential adverse effects by trying to minimize the *perceived* risks of medication by taking less. This is, after all, a logical response if one believes that the medication is necessary to control the illness yet are simultaneously concerned about potential adverse effects of taking it: one takes some but not all of the recommended dose.

For many people, adherence to medication seems to be influenced by a cost–benefit analysis in which beliefs about the necessity of their medication are weighed against concerns about the potential adverse effects of taking it. However, this does not imply that each time the patient is required to take a dose of medication, they sit down and think through the pros and cons of doing so! The 'cost–benefit analysis' may be implicit rather than explicit. For example, in some situations, non-adherence could be the result of a deliberate strategy to minimize harm by taking less medication. Alternatively, it might simply be a reflection of the fact that patients who do not perceive their medication to be important may be more likely to forget to take it (Horne *et al.*, 2004). The impact of perceptions of treatment on adherence is also likely to be influenced by beliefs about adherence, such as the importance of strict adherence to achieve the desired outcome. A key question here is 'What can I get away with?' (Siegel *et al.*, 2000).

Patients' ideas about their illness and treatment are usually related to one another in a logically consistent way. This is illustrated by considering some of the correlates of necessity beliefs and concerns.

The common-sense origins of medication necessity beliefs: symptom interpretation and perceptions of illness

We can differentiate two stages in the process by which we arrive at our views about our need for a particular treatment. First, we need to be convinced that our condition warrants treatment. Then we have to decide whether the specific treatment is the one that we need as opposed to some other.

Unsurprisingly, perceptions of need for prescribed medication are influenced by our beliefs about the illness and experience of symptoms. Over the last few decades, developments in theory and research have greatly enhanced our understanding of the psychology of illness and symptom perception. A range of theoretical models have been developed to explain how people think about health and health-threats and how psychological processes influence health-related behaviour. A detailed consideration of these models is beyond the scope of this chapter but a brief overview can be found elsewhere (Horne &

Weinman, 1998). However, one theoretical approach is particularly germane to our discussion. The self-regulatory model (SRM) developed by Howard Leventhal and colleagues focuses on how people think about and react to health threats at a cognitive and emotional level and how this affects their behaviour (Leventhal *et al.*, 1998). This theory merits attention here for two reasons. First, approaches derived from this theory have been shown to explain significant amounts of the variance in illness-related behaviour in a range of studies across illness groups and settings (Hagger and Orbell, 2003). Second, the necessity – concerns framework described earlier can be embedded within the theory to operationalize it to explain variation in adherence to medication (Horne, 2003).

The common-sense model of self regulation

The fundamental premise of the SRM (Leventhal *et al.*, 1998) is that patients respond to illness in a dynamic way based on their evaluation of the illness. People do not blindly follow health advice, even if it comes from trusted clinicians. Rather we evaluate whether following the advice makes 'common sense' in the light of our own perceptions of the illness. Understanding the process by which people make sense of health threats and how this in turn affects behaviours, such as adherence, is central to the model. The main tenets are as follows:

1 **Health threats:** these may be internal (e.g. the experience of symptoms) or external (e.g. when we are presented with a medical diagnosis or told that we are at risk of developing a disease). Either way, our first response is to build a mental map or *illness representation* that enables us to make sense of the threat and determine what to do about it.

2 **Illness representations have five components:** identity, timeline, cause, consequences, and control/cure. These can be thought of as the answers to five basic questions about the illness or health threat: What is it? How long will it last? What caused it? How will it/has it affected me? Can it be controlled or cured? Our illness representation is made up of the answers we find to these questions. Illness representations also have an emotional as well as a cognitive component. For example believing that you have a tumour may cause anxiety or depression.

3 **Symptom experiences and labels:** symptom experiences have a profound influence on illness representations. Until we experience a chronic illness most of our experience of illness is associated with symptoms and the notion of an asymptomatic illness may be counter-intuitive to many patients. Unless we have received a convincing explanation to the contrary, it may be difficult to accept that our illness has severe consequences if we experience no symptoms.

Labelling symptom experiences is an important aspect of this. Failure to achieve a convincing diagnostic label to match symptom experiences may increase anxiety and lead to repeated consultations, with the same or other practitioners, as the patient searches for a convincing diagnostic label that matches their experiences and other aspects of their representation. The process works in both directions. If our doctor diagnoses a 'silent' medical condition we search for confirmatory symptoms. This is illustrated by patients with mild hypertension who misinterpret sensations such as feeling stressed or experiencing fatigue as symptoms of high blood pressure (Pennebaker and Watson, 1988) or diabetic patients who believe that they can judge when their blood glucose is raised. Studies examining the accuracy of diabetic patients' assessment, based on symptoms, of whether their blood glucose was raised found that these were not correlated with actual blood glucose measurements (Gonder-Frederick and Cox, 1991). The point is that perceptual experiences are generally more persuasive than abstract ideas.

4 **Search for coherence:** when constructing our illness representation we try to achieve 'common-sense coherence' between the various components. For example beliefs about cause may influence perceptions of the best way to cure or control the disease. A patient experiencing chronic fatigue may find it difficult to accept that antidepressant medication or cognitive behavioural therapy presents the best option for cure or control if they believe that the fatigue is caused by a virus and are reluctant to accept that there is a 'psychological' aspect to the condition (Moss-Morris *et al.*, 1996).

5 **Representations influence action:** illness representations strongly influence our decisions about how to respond to the illness and whether or not we follow medical advice. Suggested actions that are not congruent with our illness representation are unlikely to be adopted. We may be reluctant to take prescribed medication if we believe that our illness is caused by stress that will respond to mediation or yoga.

6 **Beliefs and behaviour interact in a dynamic process and are not simply the result of a single, 'one-off', decision:** let us consider taking aspirin in response to a headache. The selection of a coping procedure (taking aspirin) is determined by beliefs about the nature of the illness threat ('My headache is stress-related and should respond quickly to aspirin'). Then this is followed by an appraisal stage in which the patient evaluates the efficacy of their coping strategy (The pain is still there 3 hours after the aspirin). If the patient appraises a particular coping strategy as being ineffective then this might result in the selection of an alternative coping strategy ('I will try a stronger pain killer') or even a change in the representation of the illness ('Aspirin hasn't worked, this might be something more serious than a headache').

7 **The role of emotion**: the fact that cognitive and emotional processing occur in parallel may be used to explain responses to illness threats which are apparently irrational. For example a patient may believe that the lump in her breast is likely to be a tumour but delays seeking help because she fears the diagnosis (Phelan *et al.*, 1992). Her behavioural response (to delay seeking help) can be seen as a way of coping with the emotion (fear/ distress) generated by the cognitive representation, which may be reinforced by her appraisal that the lump doesn't get bigger and 'the less she thinks about it the better she feels'.

How illness representations inform perceptions of treatment necessity

1 **Symptom perceptions:** initial perceptions of treatment necessity and subsequent appraisal are influenced by symptom experiences and expectations. The effect of symptom experiences on views about medication necessity may be quite complex. At one level symptoms may stimulate medication use by acting as a reminder or by reinforcing beliefs about its necessity. Conversely, the absence of severe symptoms might cause us to interpret the condition as more benign than it actually is and hence to doubt the need for treatment (Horne *et al.*, 2001a; Siegel and Gorey, 1997). Patients' expectations of symptom relief are also likely to have an important effect. This could be problematic if the expectations are unrealistic. For example a patient who expects their newly prescribed antidepressant medication to relieve their symptoms of depression after a few doses is likely to be disappointed when they find that the medication takes several days or weeks to have any effect. This might cause them to believe that the medicine is ineffective and that continued use is not worthwhile. Symptom experience may also influence medication concerns if they are interpreted by the patient as medication side-effects (Cooper, 2004), or, alternatively, as evidence that the medication is not working (Leventhal *et al.*, 1986).

2 **Illness consequences and timeline:** as the person searches for a coherent explanatory model of the illness, symptom experiences inform representations of timeline and personal consequences and also perceptions of treatment necessity (Horne and Weinman, 2002). This can be illustrated by considering two patients with asthma. The first shares the 'medical view' of asthma as an 'acute on chronic' condition (i.e. it is a chronic disease which manifests as acute symptomatic flair up or asthma attacks) with serious consequences. This patient understands that asthma remains a problem even when there are no overt symptoms of breathlessness. The rationale for the regular use of inhaled steroid (to prevent or at least lower the frequency of attacks) is easy to accept.

Contrast this with a second patient whose model of asthma is closely linked to symptom experience. This patient doesn't think that their asthma has serious consequences because their attacks happen fairly infrequently. Although they feel very ill during the asthma attack, at other times they have no symptoms. They doubt their personal need for preventative medication because the notion of asthma as a chronic condition, needing continuous treatment, is at odds with their experience of it as an episodic problem. The first patient will be more likely to agree with the *necessity* of regular prophylactic medication than the second patient, who perceives their asthma to be an acute problem (short timeline), with few personal consequences.

3 **Causal attributions:** we might expect perceptions of personal need for individual treatment options to be influenced by beliefs about the putative causes of the illness. Changing diet may be perceived to be more necessary than taking medication if the person believes that diet causes the illness. However, we have not found causal beliefs to be strongly related to medication necessity in our studies of chronic illness. This may be because we have found relatively little variation in causal beliefs between patients with the same chronic illness.

4 **Control/cure**: relationships between treatment beliefs and beliefs about illness control are specific to the type of control belief. Necessity beliefs are positively correlated with beliefs that the illness will be controlled by treatment (a form of efficacy belief) but not with other control beliefs, for example chance/fate or personal control over illness (Horne and Weinman, 2002). The relationship between beliefs about illness controllability and treatment need is conditional on the perception that the particular treatment is appropriate.

Prototypic beliefs about diseases

Bishop and Converse (1986) suggest that people have prototypic representations of common illnesses. These prototypes serve as standards against which people match and evaluate information about experienced symptoms. Prototypic beliefs about diseases are also likely to influence perceptions of treatment necessity. Patients will be less convinced of their need for treatment if their experience of symptoms and perceptions of cause, timeline, consequences, and controllability do not match expectations derived from prototypic beliefs about the illness. This point is illustrated by research investigating the reasons for patient delay in seeking treatment for acute myocardial infarction. Delay was significantly longer for patients whose prototypic beliefs about a heart attack (e.g. sudden onset of central chest pain with collapse) did not match their actual experience of the acute event (e.g. the gradual onset of more diffuse, less 'cardiac-specific' symptoms such as nausea, fever, or feeling faint) (Horne et al., 2000; Perry et al., 2001). It is also illustrated by a recent study exploring the reasons why people with HIV refused treatment with highly active antiretroviral medication (HAART). Evidence-based guidelines for the optimum time to initiate HAART stipulate CD4 count (an indicator of immune status) and viral load (a marker for disease activity) as key indicators for when HAART is clinically indicated. However, receiving 'abstract' information about personal CD4 and viral load lab results was less persuasive than more 'concrete' symptom experiences. A common reason given by interviewees for refusing HAART was that they were experiencing few, if any, of the symptoms that they associated with late-stage HIV/AIDS (Cooper et al. 2002). Their experiences (feeling fine) did not match their prototypic beliefs about when HAART would be necessary.

Perceptions of personal resilience

Determining the necessity of a treatment may also be influenced by notions of self. There has been disappointingly little research in this area, but perceptions that one can resist the progress of disease by drawing on sources of 'inner strength', 'hardiness', or by keeping a 'positive outlook' emerged as reasons for rejecting HAART in interviews with over 100 HIV-positive men (Cooper et al., 2002). At present, we know little about the role of optimistic bias in judgements about treatment outcome and hence in treatment decisions. However, given the fairly ubiquitous effect of optimistic bias in judgements about a range of other health risks (Weinstein, 1989), it is very likely that equivalent effects will be found in relation to illness and treatments.

The common-sense origins of medication concerns

Social representations of pharmaceuticals

Research has shown that many people are suspicious about medicines, perceiving them to be fundamentally harmful substances that are over-prescribed by doctors. This view is linked to wider concerns about scientific medicine, lack of trust in doctors (Calnan et al., 2004), and an increasing interest in alternative or complementary health care. People with a more negative orientation to medicines in general tend to have stronger concerns about the potential adverse effects of medication that has been prescribed for them and are consequently less adherent (Horne and Weinman, 1999).

Perceptions of specific medicines are related to more general 'social representation' of medicines as a whole (Horne et al., 1999). When asked to talk about medicines, people seem to draw on beliefs relating to medicines as a *class* of treatment sharing certain general properties (Britten, 1994; Echabe *et al.*, 1992). Many patients and student volunteers have a fairly negative view of medicines as a whole, perceiving them as generally harmful substances that are overused by doctors (Horne *et al.*, 2001b; Horne *et al.*, 1999). Moreover, the dangerous aspects of medication are often linked to their chemical/unnatural origins and greater concern about the potential adverse effects of prescribed medication (Horne *et al.*, 1999) and non-adherence (Peters *et al.*, 2001). Beliefs about medicines as a class of treatment are likely to influence a patient's expectations of a new prescription offered by the clinic, be they positive (e.g. 'I think it will help and is just what I need') or negative (e.g. 'I am likely to get side-effects or encounter problems with this treatment'). These initial expectations might influence how subsequent events are interpreted – for example whether symptoms are attributed to the illness or the treatment (Seigel *et al.*, 1999). They may even influence outcome directly through the placebo/nocebo effect.

We can only speculate on the origins of this view. One possibility is that information about a particular medicine (e.g. speculation in the press that antidepressants are 'addictive') might feed into a 'general schema' and is extrapolated to mean that 'most medicines are addictive'. Negative experiences with medicines in the past (self or significant others) are also likely to have an effect. Negative views about medicines in general appear to be related to a broader 'world view' characterized by suspicion of chemicals in food and the environment (Gupta and Horne, 2001), and the perception that complementary therapies (e.g. homeopathy/ herbalism) are more 'natural' and safer (Horne *et al.*, 1999). This appears to be related to an increasing suspicion of science, medicine, and technology within Western cultures (Horne *et al.*, 2001b; Petrie and Wessely, 2002). Suspicions of medicines, chemicals, and related 'modern health worries' are associated with the use of complementary therapies and with rejection of medication (Gupta and Horne, 2001; New and Senior, 1991; Petrie *et al.*, 2001).

Perceptions of personal sensitivity to medication

Attitudes to pharmaceuticals may be influenced not only by beliefs about their intrinsic properties and how they are used by doctors but also by perceptions of the self in relation to medicines. Beliefs about *personal sensitivity* to the effects of medication are likely to be particularly salient.

A Sensitive Soma Assessment Scale (SSAS) has recently been developed to assess beliefs about personal sensitivity to pharmaceuticals (Horne *et al*, 2004) and preliminary research with this scale has produced some interesting findings. Predictably, people who view themselves as being particularly sensitive to the adverse effects of medication have stronger concerns about their prescribed medication and tend to perceive medicines in general as intrinsically harmful and overused by doctors. Sensitive soma beliefs also influence perceptions of the amount of medication necessary to produce beneficial effects or harm and hence are related to lower rates of uptake and adherence to prescribed medication. Perceived sensitivity to medicines may also be related to the reporting of side-effects. In a study of responses to vaccination, baseline SSAS scores predicated a greater number of symptoms experienced 20 minutes after vaccination and number of symptoms attributed to vaccination. These relationships remain after controlling for negative mood and anxiety (Petrie *et al.*, 2003).

A speculative mechanism for this effect is that perceptions of personal sensitivity to medicines establish an expectation of adverse effects, making the patient more vigilant and perhaps causing unrelated symptoms to be misattributed to the medication (Pennebaker and Watson, 1988). We know little about the origins of sensitive soma beliefs, but they may arise from more general perceptions of self and hardiness and from past experiences (of self and others).

In summary then, our perceptions of the risks (and benefits) of medication (and other treatments are likely to be influenced by a range of factors including our 'prototypic' beliefs about classes of treatments, the past experiences of ourselves and others, social and cultural norms, as well as the information we receive from various sources.

Parallel processing of cognitive and emotional representations of treatment

Just as with illness representations, cognitive and emotional aspects of treatment representations are processed in parallel. Beliefs that taking medication will result in unpleasant side-effects may be a source of anxiety and worry. In some situations, such as the prescription of intensive cancer chemotherapy or radical surgery, people may fear the treatment more than the illness. They may therefore decide that it is better to reject treatment that might prolong life on the grounds that it might diminish the quality of life.

In summary, research into patients' beliefs about their illness and treatment illustrates the following key principles about the psychology of adherence:

◆ Patients' beliefs about their illness and treatment are logically coherent. Although the patient's interpretation and ideas about their illness may appear mistaken from the medical perspective, they are 'common sense' interpretations based on their own understanding and experiences.

- Patients' behaviour (e.g. taking or not taking medication) may be more strongly influenced by their own 'common-sense' interpretation of their illness and treatment than by medical advice or instructions.

- Patients' common-sense interpretation are sometimes based on potentially modifiable misconceptions about the nature of the illness and about the benefits and risks of the treatment.

Implications for research and practice

The prescribing consultation and the concept of concordance

Recently, the debate about how to respond to the problem of non-adherence has centred on the prescribing consultation as the main source of the problem and hence the best target for solutions. The concept of concordance grew from a review of the literature on treatment compliance and discussions within a committee of health-care researchers, clinicians, and managers, established by the Royal Pharmaceutical Society of Great Britain (RPSG) and funded by Merck Sharpe and Dohme Ltd (1997). This recognized the importance of patients' personal beliefs about their illness and treatment. Non-adherence was often the outcome of a prescribing process that failed to take account of the patient's beliefs, expectations, and preferences (Horne, 1998; McGavock, 1996). It could be an indicator of poor communication within the consultation. Moreover, the fault line within the consultation was the failure to recognize that patients and clinicians bring two sets of (potentially opposing) beliefs about the nature of the illness and treatment. Consultations that ignored the patient's perspective would be more likely to lead to treatment decisions that were not 'agreed' by the patient with an increased risk of non-adherence. Such consultations fail to attain concordance or a 'shared agreement about between the patient and prescriber.

It is important to recognize that concordance is not the same as adherence or compliance. Concordance descries the outcome of an interaction between patient and clinician (e.g. doctor, nurse, or pharmacist). Adherence (compliance) describes the patient's behaviour. Concordance does not necessarily guarantee adherence (concordance may be attained but the patient may still fail to take their medication because they forget or because the regimen is too complex).

The concept of concordance contributes to the adherence debate by highlighting the fact that good prescribing is a process of negotiation between patient and practitioner in which the patients' views are taken into account. However, in common with related concepts such as shared decision making and patient-centred, concordance has yet to be fully operationalized and it is not yet clear how it should be applied in practice (Dieppe and Horne, 2002). There is much to be learned about the best way to conduct prescribing consultations and the issues are complex, as can be seen from Fig. 8.1, illustrating some of the key input, process, and outcome variables that are relevant. However, given that over a third of all medicines appear to be wasted, this is a high priority for research and practice. See Horne and Weinman (2004) for more detailed discussion of this matter.

The potential tension between patient choice and evidence-based medicine

It may be too simplistic to consider the consultation in isolation. It is more than a meeting between patient and clinician. The core decision involves at least three parties: the patient, the prescriber, and the payer. A philosophy of prescribing which ignores the latter may be noble but ultimately limited in its capacity to foster pragmatic solutions to questions of how best to use medicines. Within the UK National Health Service, the prescriber is responsible for allocating resources on behalf of 'society' and the needs of the individual must be viewed in the context of the needs of others. What happens when the patient's preferences conflict with the 'greater good', for example when a patient wants to receive an expensive new medicine but the prevailing evidence suggests that the medicine will not be effective (Barber, 1995)?

This hypothetical example illustrates the potential tension between two of the prevailing ideas in the debate about the future of medicine: evidence-based medicine and patient-centred medicine. What happens when the patient's preferences conflict with the prevailing evidence? What if a patient rejects a potentially life-saving treatment (such as immunosuppressant therapy following renal transplantation) due to erroneous interpretations of the likely risks vs. benefits or because of beliefs that are factually incorrect? A similar set of questions apply in circumstances where the patient's preferences could result in harm to themselves or others.

For many illnesses and treatments the relationship between taking medication and outcome is unclear. However, in others the evidence is much stronger. In such cases it is inappropriate to advocate the primacy of the patient's decision if this is based on erroneous beliefs. Here the duty of the clinician is to promote informed choice. In cases where patients choices are informed by erroneous interpretations of the prevailing evidence (e.g. the likely risks and benefits of treatment) or on misplaced beliefs, then passively 'respecting' these

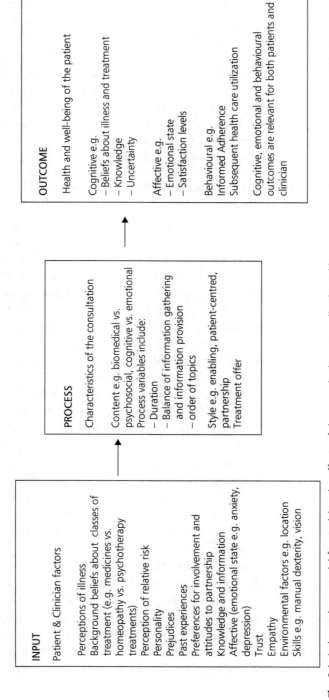

INPUT

Patient & Clinician factors

Perceptions of illness
Background beliefs about classes of
treatment (e.g. medicines vs.
homeopathy vs. psychotherapy
treatments)
Perception of relative risk
Personality
Prejudices
Past experiences
Preferences for involvement and
attitudes to partnership
Knowledge and information
Affective (emotional state e.g. anxiety,
depression)
Trust
Empathy
Environmental factors e.g. location
Skills e.g. manual dexterity, vision

PROCESS

Characteristics of the consultation

Content e.g. biomedical vs.
psychosocial, cognitive vs. emotional
Process variables include:
– Duration
– Balance of information gathering
  and information provision
– order of topics

Style e.g. enabling, patient-centred,
partnership
Treatment offer

OUTCOME

Health and well-being of the patient

Cognitive e.g.
– Beliefs about illness and treatment
– Knowledge
– Uncertainty

Affective e.g.
– Emotional state
– Satisfaction levels

Behavioural e.g.
Informed Adherence
Subsequent health care utilization

Cognitive, emotional and behavioural
outcomes are relevant for both patients and
clinician

Fig. 8.1 A three-phase model for studying the effects of the consultation on medication taking.

beliefs or 'agreeing to differ' might represent a lapse in care and duty to the patient. A more active approach is warranted where the clinician tries to identify and alter misconceptions and to challenge beliefs that appear to be incompatible with the prevailing evidence.

Informed adherence (Horne and Weinman, 2004)

The concept of concordance has contributed to the debate about the problem of non-adherence by reinforcing the importance of patients' beliefs as determinants of adherence and identifying the prescribing consultation as an important source and potential remedy of the problem. At a time when public trust in doctors and science is undoubtedly diminishing (Horton, 2003), a better understanding of patients' beliefs and preferences is clearly a priority for research and clinical practice. Prescribers have an ethical imperative to facilitate informed patient choice about whether or not to adhere to recommendations for the use of medicines and other treatments.

Michie and colleagues have outlined a model for informed choice in healthcare and this is a good starting point for discussion about informed choice in relation to adherence to medicines (Michie *et al.*, 2003). They propose that the key components of informed choice are knowledge and beliefs. The patient can be considered to have made an informed choice if they can demonstrate knowledge of relevant information about the screening test or the treatment and then act according to their beliefs.

However, in applying this framework to choice about using treatments that are supported by a strong evidence base, the clinician has a duty that goes beyond providing information. Informing should be an active process, which involves more than simply presenting the evidence. It also entails eliciting the patient's beliefs and identifying whether pre-existing beliefs might act as a barrier to an unbiased interpretation of the evidence. If the interpretation of information is influenced by misconceptions about the illness and treatment, then can the choice be truly informed?

Informed adherence should be a target for consultations in which evidenced-based medicine is used to guide initial recommendations for treatment. These are then presented to the patient in a way that takes account of their beliefs and preferences and attempts to help the patient resolve any incompatibilities between their personal beliefs and the prevailing evidence. Another important aspect of the concept is the recognition that adherence is not always a good thing. Unquestioning adherence to an inappropriate prescription (*uninformed* adherence) is clearly undesirable. A fundamental question is the degree to which the patients' (and clinicians') beliefs and preferences match the available evidence. We are still left, of course, with the problem of uncertainty in medicine. In many cases the available evidence will be inconclusive. Here the goal of the informed choice is to facilitate an interpretation of the available evidence that is unencumbered by misconceptions.

A perceptions and practicalities approach to facilitating informed adherence

We have also discussed some of the key attributes of informed adherence. Patients' beliefs about illness and treatment are key variables but we must also consider the role of information from a range of sources (e.g. medical, internet, family, friends, media), how this is interpreted by the patient, and the effect of information on knowledge and beliefs.

I have argued that patient's beliefs about medication are key to adherence decisions and have presented a simple necessity – concerns framework to show how these might be operationalized. This framework can be easily applied in practice. Clinicians can elicit a patient's perceptions of their personal need for treatment and their concerns about potential adverse effects as a basis for adherence-related discussions. Beginning with a consideration of the patient's perceptions of their need for the proposed treatment and their personal concerns about taking it would identify perceptual barriers to adherence. It would also help to foster a relationship in which the patient was able to contribute as a partner in the selection of treatment and the subsequent review of its effects.

In focusing on the role of beliefs we should not lose sight of the importance of unintentional non-adherence. For many patients the causes of non-adherence have little to do with beliefs or preferences. They may simply forget to take their medicine or encounter practical difficulties in using it. It is important to recognize this and to develop effective ways of supporting adherence by helping patients to overcome the practical barriers to regular use of medicines (e.g. by issuing reminders, by simplifying the regimen, and improving skills at using dosage devises such as inhalers).

Summary and conclusions

Good prescribing is about more than pharmacology. It is represents a compromise between two value systems: the scientific evidence base which determines the most safe and (cost) effective option for treatment and the patient's common-sense beliefs about the illness and treatment. The difficulty comes when there is conflict between these and intentional non-adherence is the result.

The concept of 'informed adherence' can be used as a guiding principle to inform solutions to the problem of non-adherence. Here, the role of the practitioner is to help ensure that the patient's decision about using medicines can be informed by a realistic assessment of the likely benefits and risks rather than by potentially misplaced beliefs or myths. To do this, practitioners will need to elicit to patients' views but also to challenge and try to change beliefs that they consider to be based on misconceptions or erroneous interpretations of the evidence.

To assist patients to self-manage chronic illness by getting the best from medicines, clinicians could adopt a Perceptions and Practicalities Approach (Horne, 2001) to facilitate informed adherence. This involves eliciting and helping to reduce both perceptual barriers (e.g. potentially misplaced beliefs about the illness and about the relative risks and benefits of treatment options) and practical barriers (e.g. poor comprehension, forgetting, regimen complexity) to appropriate adherence.

We are still left with the problem of uncertainty in medicine. Most prescribing decisions are, to some extent, therapeutic experiments. Treatment choices are guided by assumptions about likely risks and benefit based on an extrapolation of the results of group effects from clinical trials to the unique situation of the individual. The challenge for clinicians is to present the medical rationale for prescription in a way which can be understood by the patient and to identify and attempt to correct misconceptions that might act as a barrier to achieving an improved quality of life. Having done this, the patient's 'informed decision' should be respected but cannot necessarily be acted upon (e.g. if it conflicts with the greater good). Finding better ways of helping patients and clinicians to work in partnership to achieve informed adherence to evidence-based prescriptions is a priority for research and practice.

References

Arluke A (1980). Judging drugs: patients' conceptions of therapeutic efficacy in the treatment of arthritis. *Human Organization*, **39**, 84–88.

Barber N (1995). What constitutes good prescribing. *British Medical Journal*, **310**, 923–925.

Bishop GD and Converse SA (1986). Illness representations: a prototype approach. *Health Psychology*, **5**, 95–114.

Britten N (1994). Patients' ideas about medicines: a qualitative study in a general practice population. *British Journal of General Practice*, **44**, 465–468.

Calnan M, Montaner D and Horne R (2005). How acceptable are innovative health-care technologies? A survey of public beliefs and attitudes in England and Walws. *Social Sciences and Medicine*, **60**, 1937–1948.

Conner M and Norman P (1996). *Predicting health behaviour: research and practice with social cognition models*. Buckingham: Open University Press.

Cooper V, Buick D, Horne R, Lambert N, Gellaitry G, Leake H and Fisher M (2002). Perceptions of HAART among those who have declined a treatment offer: preliminary results from an interview-based study. *AIDS Care*, **14**(3), 319–328.

Coulter A (1985). Decision making and the pill: the consumer's view. *British Journal of Family Planning*, **11**, 98–103.

Dieppe P and Horne R (2002). Soundbites and patient centred care. *British Medical Journal*, **325**, 605.

DiMatteo MR (2004). Variations in patients' adherence to medical recommendations: a quantative review of 50 years of research. *Medical Care*, **42**, 200–209.

Echabe AE, Guillen CS and Ozmaiz JA (1992). Representations of health, illness and medicines: coping strategies and health promoting behaviour. *British Journal of Clinical Psychology*, **31**, 339–349.

Gabe J and Lipshitz Phillips S (1982). Evil necessity? The meaning of benzodiazepine use for women patients from one general practice. *Sociology of Health and Illness*, **4**, 201–209.

Gill A and Williams AC (2001). Preliminary study of chronic pain patients' concerns about cannabinoids as analgesics. *Clinical Journal of Pain*, **17**, 245–248.

Gonder-Frederick LA and Cox DJ (1991). Symptom perception, symptom beliefs and blood glucose discrimination in the self-treatment of insulin dependent diabetes. In: JA Skelton and RT Croyle, eds. *Mental representation in health and illness*, pp. 220–246. New York: Springer-Verlag.

Gupta K and Horne R (2001). The influence of health beliefs on the presentation and consultation outcome in patients with chemical sensitivities. *Journal of Psychosomatic Research*, **50**, 131–137.

Hagger MS and Orbell S (2003). A meta-analytic review of the common-sense model of illness representations. *Psychology and Health*, **18**, 141–184.

Hand CH and Bradley C (1996). Health beliefs of adults with asthma: toward an understanding of the difference between symptomatic and preventive use of inhaler treatment *Journal of Asthma*, **33**, 331–338.

Haynes RB, McDonald H, Garg AX and Montague P (2002). Interventions for helping patients to follow prescriptions for medications. The Cochrane Database for Systematic Reviews, 2, CD000011.

Horne R (1997). Representations of medication and treatment: Advances in theory and measurement. In: KJ Petrie and JA Weinman, eds. *Perceptions of health and illness: current research and applications*, pp. 155–188. London: Harwood Academic.

Horne R (1998). Adherence to medication: A review of existing research. In: L Myers and K Midence, eds. *Adherence to treatment in medical conditions*, pp. 285–310. London: Harwood Academic.

Horne R (2001). Compliance, adherence and concordance. In: K Taylor and G Harding, eds. *Pharmacy practice*, pp. 165–184. London: Taylor and Francis.

Horne R (2003). Treatment perceptions and self regulation. In: LD Cameron and H Leventhal, eds. *The self-regulation of health and illness behaviour*, pp. 138–153. London: Routledge.

Horne R, Buick D, Fisher M, Leake H, Cooper V and Weinman J (2004). Doubts about necessity and concerns about adverse effects: identifying the types of beliefs that are associated with non-adherence to HAART. *International Journal of STD and AIDS*, **15**, 38–44.

Horne R, Cooper V, Fisher M and Buick D (2001a). Beliefs about HIV and HAART and the decision to accept or reject HAART. *HIV Medicine*, **2**, 195.

Horne R, Frost S, Hankins M and Wright S (2001b). 'In the eye of the beholder': pharmacy students have more positive perceptions of medicines than students of other disciplines. *International Journal of Pharmacy Practice*, **9**, 85–89.

Horne R, Petrie K, Weinman J and Vincent R (2000). Patients' interpretation of symptoms as a cause of delay in reaching hospital during acute myocardial infarction. *Heart*, **83**, 388–393.

Horne R, Sumner S, Jubraj B, Weinman J and Frost S (2001c). Haemodialysis patients' beliefs about treatment: Implications for adherence to medication and fluid-diet restrictions. *International Journal of Pharmacy Practice*, **9**, 169–175.

Horne R and Weinman J (1998). Predicting treatment adherence: an overview of theoretical models. In: L Myers and K Midence, eds. *Adherence to treatment in medical conditions*, pp. 25–50. London: Harwood Academic.

Horne R and Weinman J (1999). Patients' beliefs about prescribed medicines and their role in adherence to treatment in chronic physical illness. *Journal of Psychosomatic Research*, **47**, 555–567.

Horne R and Weinman J (2002). Self-regulation and self-management in asthma: Exploring the role of illness perceptions and treatment beliefs in explaining non-adherence to preventer medication. *Psychology and Health*, **17**, 17–32.

Horne R and Weinman J (2004). The theoretical basis of concordance and issues for research. In: C Bond, ed. *A concordance reader*. Pharmaceutical Press.

Horne R, Weinman J and Hankins M (1999). The Beliefs about Medicines Questionnaire: The development and evaluation of a new method for assessing the cognitive representation of medication. *Psychology and Health*, **14**, 1–24.

Horne R, Petrie, KJ, Davis C, Diefenbach M, Leventhal H, and Leventhal E. (2004). The Sensitive soma inventory: A new measure for assessing perceptions of personal sensitivity to medicines. *International Journal of Behavioral Medicine*, **11**(supplement), 280.

Horton R (2003). The dis-eases of medicine. In: *Second opinion: Doctors, diseases and decisions in modern medicine*, pp. 1–61. London: Granta Publications.

Leventhal H, Easterling DV, Coons HL, Luchterhand CM and Love RR (1986). Adaption to chemotherapy treatments. In: BL Andersen, ed. *Women with cancer: Psychological perspectives*, pp. 172–203. New York: Springer Verlag.

Leventhal H, Leventhal EA and Contrada RJ (1998). Self-regulation, health and behavior: a perceptual-cognitive approach, *Psychology and Health*, **13**, 717–733.

Llewellyn C, Miners A, Lee C, Harrington C and Weinman J (2003). The illness perceptions and treatment beliefs of individuals with severe haemophilia and their role in adherence to home treatment. *Health Psychology*, **18**, 185–200.

McGavock H (1996). *A review of the literature on drug adherence*. London: The Royal Pharmaceutical Society of Great Britain and Merck Sharp and Dohme.

Michie S, Dormandy E and Marteau TM (2003). Informed choice: understanding knowledge in the context of screening uptake. *Patient Education and Counseling*, **50**, 247–253.

Morgan M and Watkins CJ (1988). Managing hypertension: Beliefs and responses to medication among cultural groups. *Sociology of Health and Illness*, **10**, 561–578.

Moss-Morris R, Petrie KJ and Weinman J (1996). Functioning in chronic fatigue syndrome: do illness perceptions play a regulatory role? *British Journal of Health Psychology*, **1**, 15–25.

New SJ and Senior ML (1991). 'I don't believe in needles': qualitative aspects of a study into the uptake of immunisation in two English health authorities. *Social Science and Medicine*, **33**, 509–518.

Pennebaker JW and Watson D (1988). Blood pressure estimation and beliefs among normotensives and hypertensives. *Health Psychology*, **7**, 309–328.

Perry K, Petrie KJ, Ellis CJ, Horne R and Moss-Morris R (2001). Symptom expectations and delay in acute myocardial infarction patients. *Heart*, **86**, 91–93.

Peters KF, Horne R, Kong F, Francomano CA and Biesecker BB (2001). Living with Marfan syndrome. 2. Medication adherence and physical activity modification. *Clinical Genetics*, **60**, 283–292.

Petrie KJ, Moss-Morris R, Grey C and Shaw M (2004). The relationship of negative affect and perceived sensitivity to symptom reporting following vaccination. *British Journal of Health Psychology*, **9**, 1, 101–112.

Petrie KJ, Sivertsen B, Hysing M, Broadbent E, Moss-Morris R, Eriksen HR, *et al.* (2001). Thoroughly modern worries: the relationship of worries about modernity to reported symptoms, health and medical care utilization. *Journal of Psychosomatic Research*, **51**, 395–401.

Petrie KJ and Wessely S (2002). Modern worries, new technology, and medicine. *British Medical Journal*, **324**, 690–691.

Piette JD, Wagner TH, Potter MB and Schillinger D (2004). Health insurance status, cost-related medication underuse, and outcomes among diabetes patients in three systems of care. *Medical Care*, **42**, 102–109.

Phelan M, Dobbs J and David AS (1992). 'I thought it would go away': patient denial in breast cancer. *Journal of the Royal Society of Medicine*, **85**, 206–207.

Ross S, Walker A and MacLeod MJ (2004). Patient compliance in hypertension: role of illness perceptions and treatment beliefs, *Journal of Human Hypertension*, **18**, 607–613.

Royal Pharmaceutical Society of Great Britain (1997). *From compliance to concordance; achieving shared goals in medicine taking*. London, Pharmaceutical Press.

Siegel K and Gorey E (1997). HIV infected women: Barriers to AZT use. *Social Science Medicine*, **45**, 15–22.

Siegel K, Schrimshaw EW and Raveis VH (2000). Accounts for non-adherence to antiviral combination therapies among older HIV-infected adults. *Psychology, Health and Medicine*, **5**, 29–42.

Weinman J (1990). Providing written information for patients: Psychological considerations. *Journal of the Royal Society of Medicine*, **83**, 303–305.

Weinstein ND (1989). Effects of personal experience on self-protective behaviour. *Psychology Bulletin*, **105**, 31–50.

World Health Organization (2003). *Adherence to long-term therapies: evidence for action*. Geneva: World Health Organization.

Chapter 9

Explaining unexplained symptoms: the role of beliefs in clinical management

Peter Salmon

The challenge of unexplained symptoms

The scale of the problem

Many patients who are being treated medically or surgically for physical symptoms have no physical disease. In hospital outpatient clinics, estimates of the proportion without disease range from 30 to 70 per cent (Bass, 1990; Nimnuan et al., 2001; Maiden et al., 2003). Estimates are more difficult in primary care because definitive investigations that might exclude disease are not always available. Nevertheless, doctors think that around 15 per cent of adults who attend with persistent physical symptoms have no physical disease (Peveler, 1998; Weijden et al., 2003). These figures probably underestimate prevalence because, understandably, doctors are cautious about excluding physical disease (Nimnuan et al., 2000).

Persistent medically unexplained symptoms (PMUS) are a problem for the patients who suffer them, health care systems, and doctors. Patients have as poor a quality of life as those with comparable symptoms caused by disease (Maiden et al., 2003; Smith et al., 1986; Stanley et al., 2002) and they consume health care disproportionately (Barsky et al., 2001). They attend frequently at both primary and secondary care (Gill and Sharpe, 1999; Reid et al., 2001a). In primary care they receive more than the average drug prescriptions and secondary referrals (Stanley et al., 2002). Hospital care extends even to surgery: many patients who undergo appendectomy or hysterectomy have only healthy tissue removed (Fink, 1992; Echlin et al., 2002). Doctors dislike consultations with these patients (Sharpe et al., 1994; Garcia-Campayo et al., 1998; Hahn et al., 1994; Hartz et al. 2000; Reid et al., 2001b; Steinmetz and Tabenkin, 2001), preferring consultations where they identify physical disease (Nimnuan et al., 2000). They feel powerless and frustrated in the face of physical symptoms that defy explanation or treatment (Wileman *et al.*, 2002), even to the extent of 'heart-sink' (O'Dowd, 1988).

Of course, most patients who are told by their general practitioner (GP) that their symptoms do not indicate disease seek no further care (Thomas, 1974). However, patients in whom symptoms persist can have a poor prognosis. Because there is no disease, treatment is understandably often ineffective (Kroenke and Mangelsdorff, 1989) – paradoxically, physical symptoms in primary care recover less well when disease is absent than when it is present (Craig *et al.*, 1993). Study of patients with fatigue indicates that prognosis deteriorates as symptoms persist longer. Therefore although, in primary care, at least half of patient recover, prognosis in outpatient care is worse, most remaining impaired (Joyce *et al.*, 1997; Hickie *et al.* 1999; Skapinakis *et al.*, 2003). In general, therefore, it is found that half or more of patients with PMUS remain 'ill' and distressed over 1 to 6-year follow-up periods (Reid *et al.*, 2003; Carson *et al.*, 2003; Crimlisk *et al.*, 1998; Craig *et al.*, 1993). Moreover, even where presenting symptoms improve, patients can remain ill or impaired, perhaps because of new symptoms or residual anxiety about their symptoms (Speckens *et al.*, 1996; Mayou *et al.*, 1994).

From many doctors' perspective, a simple explanation for this perplexing scenario is that patients pressure them for ineffective somatic treatment (see: Sharpe *et al.*, 1994; Armstrong *et al.*, 1991; Stevenson *et al.*, 1999; Wileman *et al.*, 2002). This is too simple, though. Doctors are clearly challenged by these patients, and attributing the problem to the patients recalls a familiar response to challenge – to blame someone else. The explanation for the mutually unsatisfactory relationship of these patients to medical care is more complex.

Dualism and reductionism in medicine

Medicine is basically reductionist; symptoms indicate diseases and doctors seek to treat diseases (Salmon, 2000; Henningsen and Priebe, 1999). It is also dualistic; physical illnesses are distinguished from mental ones and are treated by separate doctors. Patients with PMUS challenge both principles; they have symptoms but no disease and although, as we shall see, some have evidence of *psychological* needs, they present *physical* symptoms.

For several decades, medicine incorporated PMUS into its familiar dualistic and reductionist framework. It delineated 'functional' diseases that could be diagnosed purely on the basis of symptoms that patients describe, such as fibromyalgia, migraine, irritable bowel syndrome, or chronic fatigue (Table 9.1). Although diagnosed on the basis of what patients said, these were

Table 9.1 Syndromes of unexplained physical symptoms. Sometimes the fact that medicine cannot identify a disease process to explain symptoms is masked by a medical diagnosis. The following are examples of terms in common use to describe syndromes in which physical symptoms are not caused by any known physical disease

---

Systemic syndromes – symptoms are diffuse and not identifiable with specific organ systems
  Chronic fatigue/myalgic encephalomyelitis
  Gulf war syndrome
  Total allergy syndrome

Abdominal syndromes – syndromes are defined by pain localized to specific regions of the body
  Atypical chest pain
  Irritable bowel syndrome
  Non-specific abdominal pain
  Non-ulcer dyspepsia
  Pelvic pain
  Menstrual pain
  Premenstrual syndrome

Musculoskeletal syndromes – these are characterized primarily by pain and stiffness
  Lower back pain
  Fibromyalgia
  Repetitive strain injury

---

regarded as physical diseases. At the expense of circular reasoning, symptoms could then be attributed to those diseases. This view – always logically spurious – can no longer withstand the evidence. Different functional syndromes have symptoms in common, and patients with symptoms of one tend also to have symptoms of others (Deary, 1999). The variety of syndromes probably reflects medical specialization more than underlying differences between patients (Barsky and Borus, 1999; Wessely *et al.*, 1999). Therefore, at the level of primary care, patients' symptoms simply do not fall into clusters that would support the reality of these syndromes (Stanley *et al.*, 2002). It is much easier to recognize syndromes in hospital clinics, but this is after successive consultations have selected and shaped symptoms that fit that specialty.

The second way in which medicine has sought to make unexplained symptoms fit its dualistic and reductionist principles is by 'explaining' these symptoms as 'somatization', the assumption being that they express underlying depression or anxiety which the patients deny (Goldberg and Bridges, 1988). This manoeuvre preserves reductionism because symptoms are attributed to an underlying disorder, albeit a psychiatric one (Henningsen and Priebe, 1999). Similarly, it preserves the dualistic distinction of physical from mental phenomena by allowing a disease that is mental to cause symptoms that are physical. However, while evidence of depression or anxiety is common in patients with PMUS it is not ubiquitous, and is just as likely to be a consequence of the symptoms as the cause (Stanley *et al.*, 2002). Moreover, there is no evidence to support the view that presenting physical symptoms helps patients to deny emotional distress (Hotopf *et al.*, 2001).

The role of patients' beliefs

Beliefs define and shape the problem

It is not the presence of unexplained symptoms that defines this group of patients. Symptoms of this kind exist widely in community samples and only a proportion of sufferers visit their doctor, most of whom do not return (Thomas, 1974). Therefore we are unlikely to understand the problem of PMUS better by focusing on the symptoms. Instead, it is the patients' beliefs about their symptoms and what the doctor can offer that distinguish them.

It is axiomatic that patients attend a doctor, or persist in attending, because of what they believe about their needs or the doctor's ability to meet them. Indeed, patients in whom symptoms, functional impairment, and demand for health care persist tend to be those who believe or fear that their symptoms arise from physical disease or disorder (Dulmen *et al.*, 1996; Cope *et al.*, 1994; Chalder *et al.*, 2003; Wilson *et al.*, 1994; Sharpe *et al.*, 1992; Vercoulen *et al.*, 1996; Klenerman *et al.*, 1995; Fritz *et al.*, 2001). One report suggests that, within a sample of hospital outpatients selected for hypochondriacal beliefs, how healthy they feel depends more on the extent of those beliefs than on objective indicators of medical status (Barsky *et al.*, 1992). Therefore, the starting point for understanding the problem of PMUS is to understand what patients with unexplained symptoms believe about their symptoms and about the doctors from whom they seek help.

Reality, knowledge, and authority

When patients with PMUS talk about their symptoms, the most striking feature is their conviction that their symptoms are real (Peters *et al.*, 1997). This is curious; we would not expect patients with arthritis, cancer, or 'flu to emphasize that their symptoms are real. That patients with PMUS do implies, of course, that they feel that others doubt it. Indeed, patients complain that their doctors dismiss their symptoms as unreal or 'all in the mind'. As one patient explained, 'It's not bloody psychological. I'm not off me trolley. She [GP] thinks it's all in the mind' (Peters *et al.*, 1997).

From the patient's perspective, this scenario reverses the usual view of medical consultation, in which both parties regard the doctor as the expert. In fact that view is overstated, because there has been evidence for a long time that, as patients, we are more sceptical than doctors often realize. Whether we accept doctors' advice depends on whether it fits what we already believe (Hunt *et al.*, 1989; Stimson, 1974; Blaxter, 1989). In consultations about PMUS, in particular, the perception that doctors disbelieve the symptoms leaves patients feeling more expert than the doctor. Patients make other comparisons that strengthen their feeling of authority over their doctors. Doctors' imperfect information from X-rays and other tests compares poorly – in the patients' view – with the infallible evidence of patients' senses (Peters *et al.*, 1997). Similarly, the simplistic way in which, in the patients' view, doctors approach the symptoms contrasts with the 'scientific' way that patients try to understand them, by deriving and testing hypotheses about them, and by keeping an open mind about different explanations (Borkan *et al.*, 1995; Peters *et al.*, 1997). We shall see, below, problems that arise when doctors act in the mistaken belief that patients see *them* as the experts.

Beliefs about causes

There must be a cause

When patients describe their symptoms, the emphasis on their reality is closely linked to the view that, for example, 'these migraines must be from something' (Peters *et al.*, 1997). That is, there must be a cause, and establishing it is important to patients. Indeed, ideas about causes or explanations pervade their accounts, not as firm beliefs but as tentative possibilities, often incomplete and unsatisfactory to patients, who continue to search for more convincing explanations. Patients' accounts, therefore, are fluid as they seek and assess evidence – from their own observations or from other sources – with which to compare or evaluate explanations (Peters *et al.*, 1997). Like patients in general they consider multiple causes (Woloshynowych *et al.*, 1998; Stimson, 1974), and they describe experimenting to test their ideas, comparing doctors' explanations with what they already know and with non-medical sources of medical information, such as family, books, magazines, or, recently, the internet (Peters *et al.*, 1997). Although the range of causes that patients consider is therefore wide, they reflect a few themes that are seen across cultures and, within Western culture, across the centuries (Helman, 1994).

The disease entity

The concept of disease as an 'it' pervades the language of illness. Whereas the heart and lungs are parts of the body, heart disease and lung cancer imply something different; a disease entity that exists separately from the body (Salmon and Hall, 2003). A sociological view is that medicine separates disease from the individual to divert society's gaze from social causes of illness (Waitzkin, 1984). The concept of disease gives doctors power and status, too, because diseases 'belong' to doctors, inasmuch as they have the authority to diagnose and treat them. However, the discourse of disease as an 'it' extends beyond Western medicine (Harley, 1999), and has benefits for individuals as well as society. Attributing illness to something separate from the person allows individuals to be regarded – by themselves as well as others – as basically sound and healthy (Cassell, 1976; Helman, 1985). For example attributing to a disease problems such as not being able to work or meet family obligations avoids the culpability that is associated with alternative explanations, such as laziness or malingering. Moreover, once problems have been packaged in the language of disease, patients can seek to hand responsibility for managing them to the doctor (Salmon and Hall, 2003).

The way in which patients with PMUS describe their symptoms shows that they also believe that a disease underlies them (Table 9.2). Moreover, until this disease receives a benign label, it can be very frightening: as one patient explained: 'Not having a label, I think that's the main problem so I can put it in a box and go "yeah, it's that, I've got that, now I can get on with my life." ' I can't deal with the unknown' (Peters *et al.*, 1997).

Bodily imbalance

Other culturally widespread and historically persistent themes of illness causation permeate patients' accounts. That illness reflects imbalance of bodily elements is explicit in Chinese medical theories that describe the effects of

Table 9.2 The disease entity. These statements were made by patients with persistent medically unexplained symptoms (PMUS) (Peters *et al.*, 1997). They describe a disease entity with the following characteristics

Can exist outside the patient's body	'It just come on me and never left me'
Invades the body	'The glandular fever left a scar on the lung. I assume that's where the [ME: myalgic encephalomyelitis/chronic fatigue] virus got in'
Moves through the body	'The migraine starts here and moves to here'
Changes its form	'That [ME] started from glandular fever and it just turned into the ME'
Resists attack	'I'd beaten it and it came back'
Evades capture	'It's never got caught when you've gone for tests'

imbalance of Yin and Yang, just as it was in Hippocrates' theory of the humours. A diverse range of specific causal ideas evoke internal imbalance in modern Western culture (Helman, 1994). Patients with PMUS, like others, attribute illness to the immune system being weakened, to chemical imbalances, over-heating (inflammation), or to demanding more of the body than it can sustain (Peters *et al.*, 1997).

Other people

Attributions of illness to other people also cross cultures and span the centuries. Westerners, who regard attributions to witchcraft or to evil spells as primitive, readily blame illness on employers or families expecting too much of them. Thereby, the Western concept of stress evokes a global and historical tendency to blame others for illness. Stress is amongst the most common of primary care patients' explanations for symptoms (Skelton *et al.*, 2002; Woloshynowych *et al.*, 1998), and patients with PMUS also freely attribute symptoms to work, family life, or social demands (Peters *et al.*, 1997; Salmon *et al.*, 2004; Targosz *et al.*, 2001; Kirmayer and Young, 1998).

Nerves and moods

'Nerves' are blamed for illness in many cultures, including the West (Helman, 1994), and patients with PMUS share this language. The language of nerves, at least in the West, extends to linking illness to mood, including anxiety and depression and here, again, some patients with PMUS resemble other patients in linking their illness to these factors (Peters *et al.*, 1997; Salmon *et al.*, in press). PMUS patients also echo the tendency across cultures to link illness to the long-lasting effects of previous trauma (Kirmayer and Young, 1998; Waitzkin and Magana, 1997).

Metaphor in belief

It is tempting to classify attributions to stress, nerves, or mood as 'psychological' attributions, in contrast to 'physical' attributions to imbalance or a disease entity. However, to do so would be to impose medicine's dualistic framework on attributions that do not invite this categorization. In the concept of stress, for example, patients with PMUS and other symptoms interweave mechanisms in a way that transcends the distinction of physical from psychological (Peters *et al.*, 1997; Woloshynowych *et al.*, 1998). From the patients' perspective, therefore, symptoms can easily be expressions or products of psychosocial difficulties (Borkan *et al.*, 1995; Peters *et al.*, 1997), and it is professionals' concern with separating physical and psychological factors that is aberrant.

A second reason why it is pointless to categorize beliefs as physical or psychological is that they can rarely be understood 'literally' (that is in terms of their conventional meaning within medical discourse). Often patients echo medical explanations, when they use words like 'nerves', 'virus', or 'allergy'. However, as we have seen, they typically use these to refer to beliefs that are based on non-medical ideas, including culturally long-standing ones that attribute disease to, for example, invasion of the body by a disease entity or to imbalance of bodily elements. Indeed, the ways that patients use medical terms often indicate understanding of the body at variance with medical knowledge. To a large extent, patients understand their symptoms using familiar metaphors (Skelton, 2002). For example imbalance is a metaphor, as is stress. More specific metaphors are used, also. Mabek and Olesen (1997) suggested that Western patients understand the body in terms of a system of 'ethnomechanics'. For example a plumbing metaphor underlies ideas of blockage and pressure in the body, and beliefs that the body lacks energy, or that part of it is worn out, indicate a metaphor of the body as machine. Similarly, patients undergoing tests for unexplained pain (and perhaps their doctors, too) interpret those tests using a metaphor of vision: the interior of the body and all its workings and problems should be visible to the doctors through the instruments that extend the gaze of the eye (Rhodes *et al.*, 1999; Kirmayer and Young, 1998). Culturally-specific metaphors of the body and illness such as these are so ingrained that they are easily taken as literal and often more easily recognized in other cultures (Kirmayer and Young, 1998).

Of course, the use of metaphor is not restricted to patients with unexplained symptoms. We saw, above, that 'disease' is itself metaphorical; diseases are not in reality separate from the individual, but the concept of disease allows us to regard disease as belonging to the set of entities that exist outside the person. Indeed, it is possible to argue that all knowledge of the inside of the body is based on metaphor (Kirmayer, 1992). It follows that a patient's descriptions of symptoms can only be understood from his or her perspective. Where the patient describes having a 'chill', this cannot be understood literally, but only within a conceptual framework in which the body can be invaded and damaged by cold and damp. The role of metaphor is particularly important in unexplained symptoms. Although the long-standing view that these patients are somatizing emotional problems is implausible, there is evidence that many of these patients are frightened or unhappy or have family or social problems that they indicate to their doctors (Salmon *et al.*, 2004). However, the language of emotional feelings is imbued with physical metaphors, such as 'tension' or 'depression'. Therefore, it is often difficult to know whether patients are speaking physically or emotionally. For example when a patient describes feeling 'worn out' or having 'no energy' the doctor might choose to see this as physical fatigue, whereas it could as readily be regarded as a psychological problem:

loss of motivation. Similarly, when a patient with unexplained bowel symptoms describes feeling 'full of shit', he might be describing his bowels using a plumbing metaphor – or speaking metaphorically about himself (Guthrie, 1992).

The social nature of beliefs

Doctors typically regard symptoms as occurring in patients' bodies, just as psychologists locate beliefs in people's heads, or at least their minds. However, neither is so confined. Each is a social phenomenon, shaped by – and shaping – interactions with family and friends (Borkan et al., 1995; Hunt et al., 1989). For example Western culture requires that, when someone gives up normal activities, stays in bed, or stops going to work, there has to be a cause (Henningsen and Priebe, 1999). Therefore family, friends, neighbours, and colleagues will enquire, muse, and discuss until they have one, whereas those in other cultures might not find this necessary. Moreover, the cause that is arrived at determines their response. Tolerance and sympathy are the prizes of an explanation that the immune system has failed to recover from a viral infection; approbation is the price of the default explanation of indolence or malingering. That is, medical explanation is an entry requirement for the 'sick role', whereby an individual is excused normal social obligations, and patients can accept or reject explanations according to their implications for legitimizing their suffering to others (Parsons, 1951; Glenton, 2003).

What do patients seek from doctors?

This background helps to explain what patients seek from their doctors. It is natural to assume that they want cure. However, when Peters et al. (1997) interviewed patients with PMUS, it was striking that none complained about doctors' failure to cure them. Instead, they valued doctors who, they felt, had engaged in alliance against the disease by taking the symptoms seriously. Beyond this, they seek explanation. However, the explanation has to meet several needs (Salmon et al., 1999; Glenton, 2003). First, it must identify a tangible mechanism, which the patient understands as signifying that the doctor accepts that the symptoms are real. Whereas attributions to anxiety and depression can leave the patient with the view that the symptoms are being dismissed as 'all in the head', links to a virus, muscle tension, or a plausible medical diagnosis legitimate the symptoms (Table 9.3). Secondly, the patient needs to be exculpated for having the symptoms. Again, patients experience simple attributions to emotional problems as blaming them, perhaps because of the cultural view that emotional difficulties proclaim moral weakness.

Table 9.3 A failure to reassure. This GP thought that his patient's symptoms were not caused by any physical disease and tried to reassure the patient. However, what he said appeared, to the patient, to reject her symptoms,[1] and he disregarded the patient's cue to provide a better explanation.[2] The patient then escalated her presentation.[3] The GP offered to repeat the tests—even though the patient had not asked for this (Dowrick *et al.*, 2003)

P:	So I've just come for my results for the scan and blood test.
GP:	Everything looks a mystery to me at first till I consult the computer. Right, right . . . the blood tests are perhaps easier because I think they are normal.[1]
P:	That's strange.[2]
GP:	A little bit of a rise in your ESR but it's not, you know, it's not significant ESR[3] . . .
P:	I've been getting more problems
GP:	Like what?
P:	Pains in my fingers, goes from my knuckles to the tips of my fingers and then my knee and my wrist and my elbows.[3]
GP:	Well I think we ought to . . . re-do the tests in an interval because it might be that we've shot our bolt too early, pre any changes, pre changes.

Belief and explanation in consultation

Contrary to assumptions, therefore, patients with PMUS do not generally seek invasive somatic treatment from their doctors, at least in primary care (Ring *et al.*, 2004). They have more subtle needs: to have their worries and concerns validated; to have their symptoms taken seriously; and to receive convincing and exculpating explanations for symptoms. Recall, though, the negative feelings that doctors describe about these patients. Patients seeking careful and sensitive engagement from doctors who feel despondent or frustrated and wish to disengage is an inauspicious basis for an effective consultation. Indeed, doctors' usual responses to PMUS are ineffective (Morriss *et al.*, in press), and it is widely accepted that their symptomatic intervention is evidence of failure to manage these consultations appropriately. Research has identified several aspects of clinical consultation about PMUS that render it ineffective, or even counter-productive, and one aspect that has the potential to help patients.

Doctor–patient conflict

Patients with chronic pain describe medical consultation as a contest like a legal trial; they need to persuade their doctors whom, they feel, are testing them and their claims (Werner and Malterud, 2003). Accordingly, studies of consultations about PMUS in surgical outpatient clinics showed how patients' attempts to engage the doctor, and doctors' attempts to disengage, lead to consultations that are characterized by opposition (Salmon and May, 1995; Marchant-Haycox and Salmon, 1997). The parties are, in effect, in conflict. Each tries to draw the consultation into areas in which they have special authority. Patients emphasize the areas that only they can know about, in particular that their symptoms are real and that they are disrupting their lives; doctors emphasize the inside of the patient's body in asserting that they have 'looked inside' and found that everything is 'normal'. Unsurprisingly, being reassured that the body is 'normal' fails to satisfy patients who know that they have symptoms, so they persist in pressuring the doctor to do something. At one level, this is a conflict between patients who seek surgery and doctors who seek to avoid removing healthy tissue. However, the foregoing analysis of patients' and doctors' perspective invites a more considered view: that patients want to be taken seriously and have their suffering acknowledged, and that doctors wish not to engage with these patients. The setting – a surgical clinic – polarizes the conflict because surgery is the way that surgeons can show that they take problems seriously.

Collusion

It is easier to avoid such polarized conflict in primary care, where GPs have a wider range of management options, including suggesting a further consultation, and patients' beliefs are more fluid because they have not been shaped by repeated consultation and hospital investigation. Both parties work to preserve the relationship, too. Indeed, one reason why GPs offer prescriptions is to maintain good relationships with patients in the belief that this is what they seek (Stevenson et al., 1999). Overt conflict about PMUS is rare in primary care (Ring et al., 2004). Instead, a common way in which GPs respond is effectively by colluding with patients in simply providing a medical label, or sanctioning a label that the patient suggests (Salmon et al., 1999). Many doctors readily provide the disease labels that patients seek by diagnosing functional diseases, although patients are becoming more aware of the circularity of these labels. As one explained: 'IBS [irritable bowel syndrome] is what they call it when they don't know what it is' (Peters et al., 1997).

Nevertheless, this kind of collusion can satisfy two important needs for patients: it frees them from social disapproval that is associated with adopting a sick role without good cause and it indicates that the doctor accepts that symptoms are real. Collaboration between doctor and patient in the form of agreement about problem labels also provides a common script for consultation

(Stanley *et al.*, 2002). However, the risk is that doctor-patient relationships operating in this way shape, reinforce and legitimize pseudo-syndromes and become, in effect if not intentionally, collusive. Moreover, this collusion is at the expense of indicating that responsibility for managing the symptoms can be the doctor's – a view that leads to disappointment and frustration when treatment fails. Clinical communication guidelines emphasize the importance of doctor–patient agreement (Brunett *et al.*, 2001). Clearly, in PMUS, agreement may be achieved at a cost to clinical care.

Reassurance

Many clinicians think that reassurance is straightforward to administer (Kathol, 1997). Indeed, simple reassurance clearly works for most primary care patients without disease in that their symptoms recover and they do not bother the doctor further (Thomas, 1974). However, reassurance at later stages in patients' care is less straightforward (Kessel, 1979; Fitzpatrick, 1996; Warwick and Salkowskis, 1985), and evidence about the value of negative investigations in reassuring patients is mixed (Howard and Wessely, 1996). Giving normal test results in outpatient clinics, accompanied by reassurance, fails to allay many patients' worries – particularly the most worried (McDonald *et al.*, 1996; Lucock *et al.*, 1997).

Patients remain anxious because they cannot accept that a normal body can coexist with continued symptoms (McDonald *et al.*, 1996). Therefore, in patients' minds, a negative result in the absence of any other convincing explanation might mean that doctors have missed something serious or are looking in the wrong place. Furthermore, details of what doctors say, or their failure to respond to patients' detailed concerns, often invalidate attempts at reassurance (Donovan and Blake, 2000). Even where reassurance has some immediate benefit, fears tend to recur in many patients within a few months of being reassured (Fitzpatrick, 1996). In this context, doctors' actions are powerful sources of evidence and are often experienced as belying the doctor's words. Referral to a specialist, or the invitation to return if treatment does not work, may indicate to the patient that the doctor fears serious disease.

By definition, patients with PMUS are not simply reassured. Nevertheless, the attempt to reassure is the characteristic medical response. It has been argued for many years that reassurance can harm patients by increasing dependence (Warwick and Salkowskis, 1985). Additionally, given the well-known role of suggestion in shaping symptoms (Barsky and Borus, 1999), the repeated tests, investigations and treatment that patients receive in doctors' attempts to exclude disease or reassure the patient probably help to shape PMUS syndromes (Stanley *et al.*, 2002). Recent analyses of primary care consultations about PMUS have now begun to show in detail how reassurance can make things worse (Dowrick *et al.*, 2004). GPs typically dismissed the likelihood of disease, or offered simple reassurance on the basis of clinical knowledge or the authority of a negative investigation. Patients responded by providing further evidence for the importance of their problems and their need for the GP's engagement; they elaborated their symptoms, re-emphasized their uncertainty or concern or even introduced new symptoms until the doctor closed the consultation by offering tests or investigations. Perhaps this should be seen as – increasingly desperate – measures to persuade doctors to take their suffering seriously (Table 9.4).

Negative test results can also help explain the conflict and opposition that characterize many consultations. In the belief that the symptoms' cause should be visible inside the body, a negative result is perceived as disconfirming the symptom in the doctor's eyes (Rhodes *et al.*, 1999). In effect, by appearing to deny the legitimacy of the patients' complaints, doctors thereby compel patients to continue asserting them: 'if you have to prove you are ill, you can't get well' (Hadler, 1996; Glenton, 2003).

Effective explanation

These scenarios are clearly perverse; doctor and patient are joined in contest, collusion, or escalation of the problem, leading to outcomes that damage the patient and dismay the doctor. However, the research that has illuminated

Table 9.4 The importance of legitimation in explanation. Patients can accept or reject very similar explanations according to whether they convey that the doctor thinks the symptoms are real (usually by describing a physical mechanism) or the patient's fault (Peters *et al.*, 1997). For each type of explanation, below, patients' reactions indicated acceptance or rejection

Attributing symptoms to depression	'She said it's just depression. But I know what depression's like. This is physical' 'I have clinical depression. It's not normal depression. It's . . . the clinical type. The doctor explained it to me quite well actually. It's between the neurons, in these synapses. Something goes awry and that happens in clinical depression. Everything that hurts, I know that it's because of the brain cells not quite working.'
Attributing symptoms to fitness or tallness	'So the doctor doesn't think anything's wrong. He keeps saying I'm just unfit. Isn't that stupid?' 'The doctor told me that 'cause I was tall I'd always suffer from my back.'

what patients with PMUS seek from their doctors, and that we have reviewed earlier in this chapter, helps to understand what goes wrong in such consultations. Insofar as patients with PMUS have a need to feel understood and to have their suffering accepted as real, they will be dissatisfied by doctors' responses that do not engage with their concerns and beliefs. The evidence in this chapter points to the role of explanation in preventing these scenarios.

Explanations for PMUS are sometimes given as part of reassurance, but are often simplistic or not based on evidence, and contradicted by other doctors (Kouyanou *et al.*, 1997). Simple attributions to anxiety or depression are typically rejected, perhaps because patients regard them as signifying that symptoms are 'in the mind' and therefore unreal (Peters *et al.*, 1997) or that they remain the patient's responsibility (Kirmayer and Young, 1998). Some GPs and hospital doctors do, however, have better responses. In patients presenting new episodes of back pain, GP-supported information and advice can change beliefs, improve health behaviour and reduce disability (Burton *et al.*, 1999; Roberts *et al.*, 2002). However, patients with *persistent* symptoms need more elaborate approaches to changing beliefs. In secondary or tertiary care, techniques of cognitive therapy have been used, with consequent improvement in symptomatology and health-care costs and, in a proportion of patients, improvement in function and emotional distress (Kroenke and Swindle, 2000; Hiller *et al.*, 2003; Raine *et al.*, 2002), although whether cognitive therapy has any specific effect in comparison with other psychosocial treatments such as relaxation or exercise is not established (Allen *et al.*, 2002). In primary care, these techniques can also be effective (Lidbeck, 2003; Raine *et al.*, 2002), but are not generally feasible; consultations are too short for GPs to use cognitive therapy, and patients are too numerous for specialist therapists to treat. Nevertheless, the implication of the findings reviewed in this chapter is that modest changes in the ways that GPs consult with such patients could change the outcome of consultation.

The key is that the patient should believe that the GP accepts that the symptoms are real (Smith *et al.*, 2003). Careful explanations can, like medical diagnoses, exculpate patients and indicate a tangible mechanism to account for symptoms (Table 9.4), linked to patients' specific concerns (Dowrick *et al.*, 2004), but these explanations can also empower patients by indicating what they can do to help themselves, for example by changes to diet or lifestyle, by relaxation or stress-management – or by just accepting and tolerating the symptoms (Table 9.5; Salmon *et al.*, 1999). Of course, explanations have to make sense to the patient, so good ones will incorporate metaphors that patients understand, rather than medical terms that may mean little – or something that the GP does not intend (Table 9.6). In consecutive GP

Table 9.5 Explaining unexplained symptoms. From patients' perspective, doctors give patients three broad types of explanation for their medically unexplained symptoms (Salmon *et al.*, 1999). 'Empowerment' is rarest – but most effective

Type of explanation	What does the doctor do?	How can patients react?
Rejection	Suggests that nothing physical is wrong	'[GP] says its anxiety and depression. It's not bloody psychological . . . She thinks it's all in the mind'
Collusion	Accepts patient's own explanation	I said 'Have I got agoraphobia?'He said 'Yes'. I thought, 'Well why couldn't you have told me?''
Empowerment	Provides a tangible mechanism to explain the symptom Exculpates the patient for having the symptom Indicates opportunities for self-management	'[GP] explained about tensing myself up so the neck kept hurting. So I've got to relax the muscles'

Table 9.6 Metaphor in explanation. Contrast two ways that gynaecologists told patients that, despite their menstrual symptoms, no disease was present. By indicating no tangible physical mechanism that might underlie the symptoms, Mr X risks the patient thinking that he regards her symptoms as 'all in the mind'. Miss Y uses a physical metaphor that will make sense to the patient to 'explain' how symptoms can arise in the absence of disease

Mr X	'There's nothing wrong inside. We've had a look and your womb is perfectly normal.'
Miss Y	'The womb is like a finely tuned machine. Which means that the problem with your periods is one of the sort of finer control of the way your womb is working. And we know that there is a very fine hormonal control on how your womb is working and how heavy your periods are and unfortunately sometimes it tends to give up and that's when your periods tend to get too heavy.'

consultations, Skelton *et al.* (2002) showed that doctors use the metaphor of body as machine to recast symptoms that patients convey in more dramatic metaphors, perhaps thereby imposing an ordered calm on patients' turbulent experience. Patients will interpret these explanations in terms of their own mechanical view of the body (Mabeck and Olesen, 1997).

The importance of GPs providing effective explanations for PMUS has been recognized since the description, 15 years ago, of a programme for teaching GPs to help patients reattribute their symptoms to benign or emotional causes

(Goldberg *et al.*, 1989). There is preliminary evidence that patients treated by GPs trained in this way fare better than others (Morriss *et al.*, in press), and the training is now being evaluated in randomized trials. However, there is already overwhelming evidence that doctors' explanations, and their perception and management of patients' beliefs, have the potential to improve outcome. Being given a definite diagnosis when first attending with a viral infection seems to protect against developing chronic fatigue 6 months later (Cope *et al.* 1994). In irritable bowel syndrome, consultation can reduce patients' somatic attributions and increase psychosocial attributions – especially where the doctor perceives patients' beliefs accurately (Dulmen *et al.* 1995). Moreover, in the same study, patients who went on to receive least medication and consultation were those in whom doctors most accurately perceived patients' concerns (Dulmen *et al.*, 1996), and patients who improved most were those whose somatic attributions and fears changed most after consultation (Dulmen *et al.* 1997).

Conclusion

In writing about PMUS, it is easy to repeat or perpetuate previous errors that misdirected medicine's attempts to help. One is to regard patients as having the problem. Logically, the problem indicated by the label PMUS is in doctors' minds, not patients'. That is, PMUS is not a property of the patient, but refers to doctors' inability to explain symptoms. Therefore different patients might have explained symptoms or PMUS, depending on which doctor they see, as doctors differ both in what they regard as physical diseases (Fitzgibbon *et al.*, 1997) and what they regard as valid explanations. If doctors do become better able to provide explanations, then many patients would, by definition, no longer have PMUS!

It follows that it would be an error also to regard patients with PMUS as fundamentally different in their needs from other patients. Indeed, doctors' failure to satisfy these patients focuses attention on aspects of medical care, including effective engagement and explanation, which are often neglected when physical disease is being treated. Everything that has been written in this chapter about PMUS patients' needs therefore applies also to patients with explained symptoms.

A third error, invited by merely using the label PMUS, is to imply that the patients so labelled are homogeneous, an impression which is then reinforced by writing a chapter based on that label. They are as diverse as the factors that might puzzle their doctors. A few have serious physical disease that their doctors have missed. Others have physical symptoms that subside when the patient is over an emotional or social problem. Some are consciously malingering. Most, however, defy being explained in such ways. Whichever category they are in, patients' beliefs and needs are individual, and often idiosyncratic, and they need a medical response based on understanding those beliefs and needs rather than one guided by the currently influential stereotype of the demanding patient with entrenched views.

Ultimately, therefore, the problem of PMUS is unlikely to be fully addressed simply by developing new techniques and skills for treating this group. The inference from the material reviewed here is that these patients are casualties of the dualistic structure of medical care and beliefs. Therefore they need clinicians who can transcend dualism to reconcile the reality of symptoms with the absence of disease. Clinical medicine therefore needs to catch up with advances in the psychology of physical symptoms and the neurophysiology of the nervous system to recognize that symptoms require more complex explanation than simply as products of disease (Sharpe and Carson, 2001).

Acknowledgments

I am indebted to Adele Ring for help in reviewing the literature and to Caroline Gaunt for help in producing the manuscript. Work described in the chapter was supported by the UK MRC.

References

Allen LA, Escobar JI, Lehrer PM, Gara MA and Woolfolk RL (2002). Psychosocial treatments for multiple unexplained physical symptoms: a review of the literature. *Psychosomatic Medicine*, **64**, 939–950.

Armstrong D, Fry J and Armstrong P (1991). Doctors' perceptions of pressure from patients for referral. *British Medical Journal*, **302**, 1186–1188.

Barsky AJ and Borus JF (1999). Functional somatic syndromes. *Annals of Internal Medicine*, **130**, 910–921.

Barsky AJ, Cleary PD and Klerman GL (1992). Determinants of perceived health status of medical outpatients. *Social Science and Medicine*, **34**, 1147–1154.

Barsky AJ, Ettner SL, Horsky J and Bates DW (2001). Resource utilization of patients with hypochondriacal health anxiety and somatization. *Medical Care*, **39**, 705–715.

Bass CM, ed. (1990). *Somatization: physical symptoms and psychological illness*. Oxford, Blackwell.

Blaxter M (1989). The causes of disease: women talking. *Social Science and Medicine*, **17**, 59–69.

Borkan J, Reis S, Hermoni D and Biderman A (1995). Talking about the pain: a patient-centred study of low back pain in primary care. *Social Science and Medicine*, **40**, 977–988.

Brunett PH, Campbell TL, Cole-Kelly K, *et al.* (2001). Essential elements of communication in medical encounters: The Kalamazoo consensus statement. *Academic Medicine*, **76**, 390–393.

Burton AK, Waddell G, Tillotson K and Summerton N (1999). Information and advice to patients with back pain can have a positive effect: a randomised controlled trial of a novel educational booklet in primary care. *Spine,* **24,** 2484–2491.

Carson AJ, Best S, Postma K, Stone J, Warlow C and Sharpe M (2003). The outcomes of neurology outpatients with medically unexplained symptoms: a prospective cohort study. *Journal of Neurology Neurosurgery and Psychiatry,* **74,** 897–900.

Cassell EJ (1976). Disease as an 'it': concepts of disease revealed by patients' presentation of symptoms. *Social Science and Medicine,* **27,** 143–146.

Chalder T, Godfrey E, Ridsdale L, King and Wessely S (2003). Predictors of outcome in a fatigued population in primary care following a randomised controlled trial. *Psychological Medicine,* **33,** 283–287.

Cope H, David A, Pelosi A and Mann A (1994). Predictors of chronic 'postviral' fatigue. *Lancet,* **344,** 864–868.

Craig TKJ, Boardman AP, Mills K, Daly-Jones O and Drake H (1993). The South London Somatisation Study I: longitudinal course and the influence of early life experiences. *British Journal of Psychiatry,* **163,** 579–588.

Crimlisk HL, Bhatia K, Cope H, David A, Marsden CD and Ron MA (1998). Slater revisited: 6-year follow up study of patients with medically unexplained symptoms. *British Medical Journal,* **316,** 582–586.

Deary IJ (1999). A taxonomy of medically unexplained symptoms. *Journal of Psychosomatic Research,* **47,** 51–59.

Donovan JL and Blake DR (2000). Qualitative study of interpretation of reassurance among patients attending rheumatology clinics: 'just a touch of arthritis, doctor?' *British Medical Journal,* **320,** 541–544.

Dowrick CF, Ring A, Humphris GM and Salmon P (2004). Normalisation of unexplained symptoms by general practitioners: a functional typology. *British Journal of General Practice,* **54,** 165–170.

Dulmen van AM, Fennis JFM, Mokkink HGA and Bleijenberg G (1995). Doctor-dependent changes in complaint-related cognitions and anxiety during medical consultations in functional abdominal complaints. *Psychological Medicine,* **25,** 1011–1018.

Dulmen van AM, Fennis JFM, Mokkink HGA and Bleijenberg G (1996). The relationship between complaint-related cognitions in referred patients with irritable bowel syndrome and subsequent health care seeking behaviour in primary care. *Family Practice,* **13,** 12–17.

Dulmen van AM, Fennis JFM, Mokkink HGA, Velden van der HGM and Bleijenberg G (1997). Persisting improvement in complaint-related cognitions initiated during medical consultations in functional abdominal complaints. *Psychological Medicine,* **27,** 725–729.

Echlin D, Garden A and Salmon P (2002). Listening to patients with unexplained menstrual symptoms: what do they tell the gynaecologist? *British Journal of Obstetrics and Gynaecology,* **109,** 1335–1340.

Fink P (1992). Surgery and medical treatment in persistent somatizing patients. *Journal of Psychosomatic Research,* **36,** 439–447.

Fitzgibbon EJ, Murphy D, OShea K, *et al.* (1997). Chronic debilitating fatigue in Irish general practice: a survey of general practitioners' experience. *British Journal of General Practice,* **7,** 618–622.

Fitzpatrick R (1996). Telling patients there is nothing wrong. *British Medical Journal,* **313**, 311–312.

Fritz JM, George SZ and Delitto A (2001). The role of fear-avoidance beliefs in acute low back pain: relationships with current and future disability and work status. *Pain,* **94**, 7–15.

Garcia-Campayo J, Sanz-Carrillo C, Yoldi-Elcid A, Lopez-Aylon R and Monton C (1998). Management of somatisers in primary care: are family doctors motivated? *Australian and New Zealand Journal of Psychiatry,* **32**, 528–533.

Gill D and Sharpe M (1999). Frequent consulters in general practice: a systematic review of studies of prevalence, associations and outcome. *Journal of Psychosomatic Research,* **47**, 115–130.

Glenton C (2003). Chronic back pain sufferers – striving for the sick role. *Social Science and Medicine,* **57**, 2243–2252.

Goldberg D and Bridges K (1988). Somatic presentations of psychiatric illness in primary care settings. *Journal of Psychosomatic Research,* **32**, 137–144.

Goldberg D, Gask L and O'Dowd T (1989). The treatment of somatisation: teaching techniques of reattribution. *Journal of Psychosomatic Research,* **33**, 689–695.

Guthrie E (1992). The management of medical out-patients with non-organic disorders: the irritable bowel syndrome. In: F Creed, R Mayou and A Hopkins, eds. *Medical symptoms not explained by organic disease,* pp. 60–69. London: Royal College of Psychiatrists and Royal College of Physicians.

Hadler NM (1996). If you have to prove you're ill, you can't get well: the object lesson of fibromyalgia. *Spine,* **21**, 2397–2400.

Hahn SR, Thompson KS, Willis TA, Stern V and Budner NS (1994). The difficult doctor-patient relationship: Somatization, personality and psychopathology. *Journal of Clinical Epidemiology,* **47**, 647–657.

Harley D (1999). Rhetoric and the social construction of sickness and healing. *Social History of Medicine,* **12**, 407–435.

Hartz A J, Noyes R, Bentler SE, Damiano PC, Willard JC and Momany ET (2000). Unexplained Symptoms in primary care: perspectives of doctors and patients. *General Hospital Psychiatry,* **22**, 144–152.

Helman CG (1985). Psyche, soma, and society: the social construction of psychosomatic disorders. *Culture and Medicine in Psychiatry,* **9**, 1–26.

Helman CG (1994). *Culture health and illness,* 3rd edn. Oxford: Butterworth.

Henningsen P and Priebe S (1999). Modern disorders of vitality: the struggle for legitimate incapacity. *Journal of Psychosomatic Research,* **46**, 209–214.

Hickie I, Koschera A, Hadzi-Pavlovic D, Bennett B and Lloyd A (1999). The temporal stability and co-morbidity of prolonged fatigue: a longitudinal study in primary care. *Psychological Medicine,* **29**, 855–861.

Hiller W, Fichter MM and Rief W (2003). A controlled treatment study of somatoform disorders including analysis of healthcare utilization and cost-effectiveness. *Journal of Psychosomatic Research,* **54**, 369–380.

Hotopf M, Wadsworth M and Wessely S (2001). Is 'somatisation' a defense against the acknowledgment of psychiatric disorder? *Journal of Psychosomatic Research,* **50**, 119–124.

Howard LM and Wessely S (1996). Reappraising reassurance – the role of investigations. *Journal of Psychosomatic Research*, **41**, 307–311.

Hunt LM, Jordan B and Irwin S (1989). Views of what's wrong: diagnosis and patients' concepts of illness. *Social Science and Medicine*, **28**, 945–956.

Joyce J, Hotopf M and Wessely S (1997). The prognosis of chronic fatigue and chronic fatigue syndrome: a systematic review. *Quarterly Journal of Medicine*, **90**, 223–233.

Kathol RG (1997). Reassurance therapy: what to say to symptomatic patients with benign or non-existent disease. *International Journal of Psychiatry in Medicine*, **27**, 173–180.

Kessel N (1979). Reassurance. *Lancet*, **I**, 1128–1133.

Kirmayer LJ (1992). The body's insistence on meaning: metaphor as presentation and representation in illness experience. *Medical Anthropology Quarterly*, **6**, 323–346.

Kirmayer LJ and Young A (1998). Culture and somatization: clinical, epidemiological, and ethnographic perspectives. *Psychosomatic Medicine*, **60**, 420–430.

Klenerman L, Slade PD, Stanley IM, *et al.* (1995). The prediction of chronicity in patients with an acute attack of low back pain in a general practice setting. *Spine*, **20**, 478–484.

Kouyanou K, Pither CE and Wessely S (1997). Iatrogenic factors and chronic pain. *Psychological Medicine*, **59**, 597–604.

Kroenke K and Mangelsdorff D (1989). Common symptoms in ambulatory care: incidence, evaluation, therapy, and outcome. *American Journal of Medicine*, **86**, 262–266.

Kroenke K and Swindle R (2000). Cognitive-behavioral therapy for somatization and symptom syndromes: a critical review of controlled clinical trials. *Psychotherapy and Psychosomatics*, **69**, 205–215.

Lidbeck J (2003). Group therapy for somatization disorders in primary care: maintenance of treatment goals of short cognitive-behavioural treatment one-and-a-half-year follow-up. *Acta Psychiatrica Scandinavica*, **107**, 449–456.

Lucock MP, Morley S, White C and Peake MD (1997). Responses of consecutive patients to reassurance after gastroscopy: results of a self-administered questionnaire survey. *British Medical Journal*, **315**, 572–575.

Mabeck CE and Olesen F (1997). Metaphorically transmitted diseases. How do patients embody medical explanations? *Family Practice*, **14**, 271–278.

Maiden NL, Hurst NP, Lochead A, Carson AJ and Sharpe M (2003). Medically unexplained symptoms in patients referred to a specialist rheumatology service: prevalence and associations. *Rheumatology*, **42**, 108–112.

Marchant-Haycox S and Salmon P (1997). Patients' and doctors' strategies in consultations with unexplained symptoms: interactions of gynecologists with women presenting menstrual symptoms. *Psychosomatics*, **38**, 440–450.

Mayou R, Bryant B, Forfar C and Clark D (1994). Non-cardiac chest pain and benign palpitations in the cardiac clinic. *British Heart Journal*, **72**, 548–553.

McDonald IG, Daly J, Jelinek VM, Panetta F and Gutman JM (1996). Opening Pandora's box: the unpredictability of reassurance by a normal test result. *British Medical Journal*, **313**, 329–332.

Morriss R, Gask L, Dowrick C, Salmon P and Peters S (in press). Reattribution and other family doctor delivered management approaches to persistent medically unexplained symptoms. In: G Lloyd and E Guthrie, eds. *Handbook of liaison psychiatry*. Cambridge: Cambridge University Press.

Nimnuan C, Hotopf M and Wessely S (2000). Medically unexplained symptoms: how often and why are they missed? *Quarterly Journal of Medicine*, **93**, 21–28.

Nimnuan C, Hotopf M and Wessely S (2001). Medically unexplained symptoms: an epidemiological study in seven specialties. *Journal of Psychosomatic Research*, **51**, 361–367.

O'Dowd TC (1988). Five years of heartsink patients in general practice. *British Medical Journal*, **297**, 528–530.

Parsons T (1951). Illness and the role of the physician: a sociological perspective. *American Journal of Orthopsychiatry*, **21**, 452–460.

Peters S, Stanley I, Rose M and Salmon P (1997). Patients with medically unexplained symptoms: sources of patients' authority and implications for demands on medical care. *Social Science and Medicine*, **46**, 559–565.

Peveler R (1998). Understanding medically unexplained physical symptoms: faster progress in the next century than in this. *Journal of Psychosomatic Research*, **45**, 93–97.

Raine R, Haines A, Sensky T, Hutchings A, Larkin K and Black N (2002). Systematic review of mental health interventions for patients with common somatic symptoms: can research evidence from secondary care be extrapolated to primary care? *British Medical Journal*, **325**, 1–11.

Reid S, Crayford T, Patel A, Wessely S and Hotopf M (2003). Frequent attenders in secondary care: a 3-year follow-up study of patients with medically unexplained symptoms. *Psychological Medicine*, **33**, 519–524.

Reid S, Wessely S, Crayford T and Hotopf M (2001a). Medically unexplained symptoms in frequent attenders of secondary health care: retrospective cohort study. *British Medical Journal*, **322**, 1–4.

Reid S, Whooley D, Crayford T and Hotopf M (2001b). Medically unexplained symptoms: General practitioners' attitudes towards their cause and management. *Family Practice*, **18**, 519–523.

Rhodes LA, McPhillips-Tangum CA, Markham C and Klenk R (1999). The power of the visible: the meaning of diagnostic tests in chronic back pain. *Social Science and Medicine*, **48**, 1189–1203.

Ring A, Dowrick C, Humphris G and Salmon P (2004). Do patients with unexplained physical symptoms pressure GPs for somatic treatment? A qualitative study. *British Medical Journal*, **328**, 1057–1060.

Roberts L, Little P, Chapman J, Cantrell T, Pickering R and Langridge J (2002). The Back Home Trial: general practitioner supported leaflets may change back pain behavior. *Spine*, **27**, 1821–1828.

Salmon P (2000). *Psychology of medicine and surgery: a guide for psychologists, counsellors, nurses and doctors.* Chichester: Wiley.

Salmon P and Hall GM (2003). Patient empowerment and control: a psychological discourse in the service of medicine. *Social Science and Medicine*, **57**, 1969–1980.

Salmon P and May C (1995). Patients' influence on doctors' behaviour: a case study of patient strategies in somatization. *International Journal of Psychiatry in Medicine*, **25**, 319–329.

Salmon P, Dowrick CF, Ring A and Humphris GM (2004). Voiced but unheard agendas: qualitative analysis of the psychosocial cues that patients with unexplained symptoms present to general practitioners. *British Journal of General Practice*, **54**, 171–176.

Salmon P, Peters S and Stanley I (1999). Patients' perceptions of medical explanation for somatisation disorders: qualitative analysis. *British Medical Journal*, 318, 372–376.

Sharpe M and Carson A (2001). 'Unexplained' somatic symptoms, functional syndromes, and somatization: do we need a paradigm shift? *Annals of Internal Medicine*, 134, 926–930.

Sharpe M, Hawton K, Seagroatt V and Pasvol G (1992). Follow up of patients presenting with fatigue to an infectious diseases clinic. *British Medical Journal*, 305, 147–152.

Sharpe M, Mayou R, Seagroatt V, Surawy C, Warwick H, Bulstrode C, *et al.* (1994). Why do doctors find some patients difficult to help? *Quarterly Journal of Medicine*, 87, 187–193.

Skapinakis P, Lewis G and Mavreas V (2003). One-year outcome of unexplained fatigue syndromes in primary care: results from an international study. *Psychological Medicine*, 33, 857–866.

Skelton JR, Wearn AM and Hobbs FDR (2002). A concordance-based study of metaphoric expressions used by general practitioners and patients in consultation. *British Journal of General Practice*, 52, 114–118.

Smith G, Monson R and Ray D (1986). Patients with multiple unexplained symptoms: their characteristics, functional health, and health care utilization. *Archives of Internal Medicine*, 146, 69–72.

Smith RC, Lein C, Collins C, *et al.* (2003). Treating patients with medically unexplained symptoms in primary care. *Journal of General Internal Medicine*, 18, 478–489.

Speckens AEM, van Hemert AM, Bolk JH, Rooijmans HGM and Hengeveld MW (1996). Unexplained physical symptoms: outcome, utilization of medical care and associated factors. *Psychological Medicine*, 26, 745–752.

Stanley IM, Peters S and Salmon P (2002). A primary care perspective on prevailing assumptions about persistent medically unexplained physical symptoms. *International Journal of Psychiatry in Medicine*, 32, 125–140.

Steinmetz D and Tabenkin H (2001). The difficult patient as perceived by family physicians. *Family Practice*, 18, 495–500.

Stevenson FA, Greenfield SM, Jones M, Nayak A and Bradley CP (1999). GPs' perceptions of patient influence on prescribing. *Family Practice*, 16, 255–261.

Stimson GV (1974). Obeying doctors' orders: a view from the other side. *Social Science and Medicine*, 8, 97–104.

Targosz SA, Kapur N and Creed F (2001). Medically unexplained symptoms, illness perception and childhood experience in neurology outpatients. *Irish Journal of Psychological Medicine*, 18, 16–20.

Thomas KB (1974). Temporarily dependent patients in general practice. *British Medical Journal*, 268, 625–626.

Vercoulen JH, Swanink CM, Fennis JF, Galama JM, van der Meer JW and Bleijenberg G (1996). Prognosis in chronic fatigue: a prospective study on the natural course. *Journal of Neurology Neurosurgery and Psychiatry*, 60, 489–494.

Waitzkin H (1984). The micropolitics of medicine: a contextual analysis. *International Journal of Health Services*, 14, 339–378.

Waitzkin H and Magana H (1997). The black box in somatization: unexplained physical symptoms, culture and narratives of trauma. *Social Science and Medicine*, 45, 811–825.

Warwick H and Salkovskis P (1985). Reassurance. *British Medical Journal*, **290**, 1028–1029.

Weijden van der T, Velsen van M, Dinant G-J, Hasselt van CM and Grol R (2003). Unexplained complaints in general practice: prevalence, patients' expectations, and professionals' test-ordering behavior. *Medical Decision Making*, **23**, 226–231.

Werner A and Malterud K (2003). It is hard work behaving as a credible patient: encounters between women with chronic pain and their doctors. *Social Science and Medicine*, **57**, 1409–1419.

Wessely S, Nimnuan C and Sharpe M (1999). Functional somatic syndromes: one or many? *Lancet*, **354**, 936–939.

Wileman L, May C and Chew-Graham CA (2002). Medically unexplained symptoms and the problem of power in the primary care consultation: a qualitative study. *Family Practice*, **19**, 178–182.

Wilson A, Hickie I, Lloyd A, *et al.* (1994). Longitudinal study of outcome of chronic fatigue syndrome. *British Medical Journal*, **308**, 756–759.

Woloshynowych M, Valori R and Salmon P (1998). General practice patients' beliefs about their symptoms. *British Journal of General Practice*, **48**, 885–889.

Chapter 10

Beliefs and obstacles to recovery in low back pain

A. Kim Burton, Gordon Waddell, and
Chris J. Main

By way of introduction

Viewed from a biological perspective, pain has a protective function, triggering escape from aversive, and possibly dangerous, stimuli. It is reasonable to view this initially in terms of an instinctive process; as the infant develops and makes sense of its world, it develops views about the nature of bodily sensation, including pain. Through processes of social learning it comes to make progressively finer discrimination between aspects of the environment and to develop complex patterns of behavioural responses. With the development of anticipation, fears and patterns of avoidance become established. With maturation, and experience in a wider range of social contexts, a complex network of beliefs, emotional responses, and pain behaviours can develop. The power of beliefs can most clearly be seen in the chronic pain patient. High levels of distress and dysfunctional avoidance behaviour is frequently accompanied by distorted beliefs and appraisals, of which the most powerful appear to mistaking 'hurt' and 'harm', and 'catastrophizing' about what the future holds. These patients may require 'heavy-duty' interventions found in interdisciplinary pain management programmes (Main and Spanswick, 2000), in which modification of disadvantageous beliefs is a major component.

More recently, though, it has been recognized that mistaken, inappropriate, or unhelpful beliefs may play a role in the persistence of pain and how we adapt to it (Pincus and Morley, 2002). Importantly, beliefs can be viewed as potential obstacles to recovery, which can be addressed using a lighter touch with a simple and clear educational approach rather than a complicated psychological intervention.

In this chapter we address beliefs about back pain from an evidence-based perspective, focusing in particular on recent initiatives designed specifically to target beliefs.

Some epidemiology

Low back pain is common and not confined to any particular demographic group, with a lifetime prevalence of 60 to 80 per cent. Children experience back pain less than adults, but by adolescence the lifetime prevalence exceeds 50 per cent (Balagué et al., 2003). Back pain remains almost as common postretirement, even if it has had less attention because it no longer impacts on work. Thus, back pain is a recurrent phenomenon at all ages, but back-related disability is uncommon before adulthood (Jones et al., 2004) and is most important during the working years of life. Clinical series have revealed that some 75 per cent of patients presenting for health care will have some persistent or recurrent pain and/or disability at 1 to 4 years follow-up (Croft et al., 1998; Burton et al., 2004). However, population studies show that at least half of all 'episodes' do not present for health care (Waxman et al., 1998), and the majority of episodes among workers do not result in workloss. Back pain can be the presenting symptom of a variety of disease processes, or due to some local pathology, but the vast majority of back pain is not associated with any identifiable pathology or injury – and is better described as 'non-specific low back pain' or 'simple backache' (Royal College of General Practitioners, 1999).

The traditional concept of back pain being categorized temporally into acute, subacute, and chronic presentations is now being challenged. Rather it manifests as 'a chronic problem with an untidy pattern of grumbling symptoms and periods of relative freedom from pain and disability interspersed with acute episodes, exacerbations and recurrences' (Croft et al., 1998). Essentially, the nature and pattern characterizes what have variously been termed 'subjective health complaints' (Ursin, 1997), 'medically unexplained symptoms' (Page and Wessely, 2003) or 'regional [pain] disorders' (Hadler, 2001).

This all calls into question the notion that back pain is due to injury, particularly work-related injury. A simple injury model alone would suggest that the risk of injury is related to exposure to physical stressors, that continued exposure will lead to further damage, and that at some stage damage will exceed repair leading to disability. It is now clear that this model does not explain the majority of back pain. Despite substantial reductions in the exposure to physical labour in developed countries, the prevalence of back pain has remained more or less unchanged, while the extent of disability (evidenced by sickness absence, workers compensation, and social security claims) increased greatly during the latter part of the twentieth century (Waddell, 2004).

Back pain, then, remains a challenge in terms both of understanding and management. This is related, in part, to its variable impact on individuals.

Some people experience little or no disabling consequences, whilst others with indistinguishable clinical presentations become crippled. Looking at workers, some will take frequent short absences, a few will take prolonged absence, whilst fewer still will drift to long-term incapacity. This latter group, though a minority, represents a large number that is costly for society. The reasons for disability associated with back pain are complex, but it is now clear that beliefs play a substantial part in feeding the process (Main and Waddell, 2004).

A little on beliefs

Beliefs are basic and relatively stable ideas about the nature of reality, which help people to understand their lives and experiences. Beliefs, along with associated attitudes, shape perceptions of what a situation or experience means to the individual, and it follows that beliefs drive behaviours. Some beliefs are very general in nature, whilst others are very specific to a particular situation. In respect of back pain, beliefs determine the perception of what has gone wrong, of what caused the pain, and its likely severity and impact on life. Beliefs are central to what people then do about their experience of back pain; about whether to rest, about whether to seek treatment, about whether to work, and about what it means for the future. Since beliefs can be, and often are, inaccurate, the behaviour they determine may be inappropriate or frankly harmful.

Beliefs are shaped from childhood onwards, being the product of experience, learning, and culture. However, as shown in Table 10.1, the sources of information that lead to beliefs about back pain are not always to be trusted. These sources interact, and an inaccurate set of beliefs generated by one source can readily

Table 10.1 Some sources of beliefs about back pain, and the potentially detrimental characteristics that can influence their accuracy

Source	Characteristics potentially contributing to inaccuracy
Family	Tendency to be over-concerned and overprotective
Medical professionals	Unreliable – different health professionals give different information and advice
Culture	Inherently inaccurate, being contaminated by outdated notions and information
Media	Sensational presentations, owing more to the need to entertain than impart information
Legislation	Inappropriate messages about health and safety, with a stimulus to enter litigation
Science	Inaccessible to most and not universally trusted

influence another. Any apparent concordance between sources is likely to strengthen inaccurate beliefs, which may then persist despite contrary experience. The world of science, in principle, should influence the other sources to engender accurate and helpful sets of beliefs, but has limited success in dispelling the myths about back pain.

Myths about back pain

Seven myths about the care and consequences of low back pain were identified by Deyo in the US and appear equally relevant in the UK (Deyo, 1998). These myths represent commonly held beliefs about the nature of back pain held by the general population, and the medical profession, during the latter part of the twentieth century – despite scientific evidence to the contrary. Table 10.2 lists the myths along with brief comments on the

Table 10.2 Seven myths about low back pain (abridged from Deyo 1998)

Myth	Reality
1 If you have a slipped disc you must have surgery: surgeons agree about exactly who needs surgery	The majority of disc problems resolve without surgery; surgery rates vary dramatically from country to country and surgeon to surgeon
2 X-ray and newer imaging tests (CT and MRI scans) can always identify the cause of pain	Scans cannot determine the source of back pain; degenerative changes on scans are mostly normal, age-related changes
3 If your back hurts, you should take it easy until the pain goes away	Staying active or returning to activity (including work), even if still painful, enhances recovery
4 Most back pain is caused by heavy lifting	The cause is mostly unknown, and the onset does not usually follow lifting; back pain is similarly common among sedentary and manual workers
5 Back pain is usually disabling	Most episodes of back pain recover uneventfully within days or weeks; few patients are disabled beyond a few days
6 Everyone with back pain should have a spine X-ray	Scan findings do not correlate with symptoms, and do not provide a reliable guide to treatment
7 Bed rest is the mainstay of therapy	Bed rest as a treatment is anathema – it interferes with staying active and leads to longer time from work

reality of the situation pertinent to each. There are many other specific beliefs, similarly inaccurate, but these seven cover a range of factors that influence what people with back pain might do as a result of holding such beliefs. Moreover, they are often iatrogenic; clinicians who promulgate these beliefs can adversely affect their patients' recovery and affect their long-term health.

A Norwegian study found that Deyo's myths remained common among the general population in 2001 (Ihlebæk and Eriksen, 2003). Around 50 per cent of people believed that that back pain was caused by lifting, that scans could identify the source of pain and were needed for diagnosis, and that surgery was needed for a disc problem. A quarter of people believed that back pain was usually disabling and that they should take it easy until the pain has gone. These researchers also looked at the same myths among general practitioners and physiotherapists (Ihlebæk and Eriksen, 2004), concluding that in Norway the seven myths are dead and buried among clinicians. This is mirrored in the UK, where General Practitioners (GP) were found to disagree with a similar set of myth statements (Chaudhary et al., 2004). Interestingly, however, a UK population study found that there were, in general, more misconceptions among people who had seen their GP than among those who had not seen a GP (Moffett et al., 2000). There may be some self-selection among those who seek health care, but it is also possible that doctors, despite what they believe in theory, either do not communicate these beliefs or fail to shift the beliefs of their patients.

These cultural myths are just examples of the sort of beliefs that people hold about back pain that can detrimentally influence their behaviour in response to that pain. Specifically, patients may have a number of fears, such as concerns about damage that may have occurred already, concern about the risk of future damage, concern about the inevitable consequences of the pain, fear that movement will make matters worse, and fear of underlying (undetected) serious disease (Von Korff and Moore, 2001; Symonds et al., 1996). Perceptions about the nature of the condition can readily translate into behaviours that may be unhelpful, such as unwarranted care seeking, demands for investigations, ceasing work, and avoiding activity, all of which can have detrimental psychological consequences. It has been suggested, in view of these misconceptions about back pain, that recovery from an acute episode is an active process that involves correction of beliefs about harm, about the need to restrict activity, and about diagnosis and cure. It is argued that community actions to correct back pain myths should be useful to prevent the development of long-term disability (Goubert et al., 2004).

Obstacles to recovery – the role of beliefs

Recovery from low back pain is generally to be expected. Most episodes settle uneventfully with or without formal health care (at least enough to return to most normal activities). Most people remain at work, and the large majority of those who do take sickness absence manage to return to work quite quickly (even if still with some symptoms). Most people with back pain are 'essentially whole people' with a manageable health problem; given the right care, support, and encouragement long-term incapacity is not inevitable.

Obviously, some people, with some episodes, do not recover and return to work, and instead go on to long-term incapacity. But if recovery is normally to be expected and the health condition *per se* does not explain failure to recover, this reverses the question – it is not so much what makes some people develop long-term incapacity, but why do some people with back pain do not recover as expected?

The development of long-term incapacity is a process in which biopsychosocial factors, separately and in combination, aggravate and perpetuate disability. Crucially, these factors can also act as obstacles to recovery and return to work. The logic of back pain management then shifts from provision of more or better health care to addressing factors that delay or prevent expected recovery. Thus, management of back pain must specifically address and overcome those factors that act as obstacles to recovery (Burton and Main, 2000; Marhold *et al.*, 2002). Obstacles are potential targets for intervention and may be turned into positive opportunities to facilitate return to work.

In clinical practice, the concept of 'obstacles' started from factors that predict chronic pain and disability, and largely focused on psychological factors. Whilst psychological obstacles to recovery can also act as obstacles to return to work, they are only part of the picture. Social security studies have focused more on social barriers to work (Waddell and Burton, 2004).

Biological, psychological, and social obstacles to return to work all appear to be important (Table 10.3), accepting that there is overlap and interaction between the different dimensions, and that their relative importance may vary in different individuals and settings and over time (Moon, 1996). Individual assessment of potential obstacles may permit a problem-oriented approach that can: (1) guide clinical evaluation; (2) identify obstacles to recovery/return to work; (3) develop targeted interventions to overcome these obstacles; and (4) facilitate rehabilitation interventions (Feuerstein and Zastowny, 1999).

Biological obstacles

The main biological obstacle is the health condition, but for back pain this should not be insurmountable, given proper clinical management. Symptoms

Table 10.3 Biopsychosocial obstacles to return to work (from Waddell and Burton, 2004, with permission)

	Obstacles to return to work
Biological	Health condition (and health care) Physical and mental capacity and activity level -v- demands of work
Psychological	Personal perceptions, beliefs and behaviour (especially about work) Psychosocial aspects of work
Social	Organizational and system obstacles Attitudes to health and disability

are often felt to be the major issue, but the correlation between pain and impairment, disability, or incapacity for work is low. Moreover, symptoms are by definition subjective and therefore at least partly a matter of perceptions.

It is traditionally assumed that the health problem is the obstacle and health care the solution, but sometimes health care may become an obstacle instead. Many observers have identified waiting list delays for consultation or treatment as one of the most potent obstacles to return to work. Inappropriate health care for back pain, particularly if combined with unhelpful medical information and advice (Hamonet *et al.*, 2001), may not only be ineffective but may block more appropriate management and return to work. The role of health professionals should be to help restore self-esteem and confidence; if, instead, the professional encounter undermines them further that will be counter-productive.

Personal/psychological obstacles

Personal/psychological factors are central to incapacity associated with back pain and they are also important obstacles to return to work. They were originally described as 'yellow flags' for risk of chronic pain and disability and unfavourable clinical outcomes (Kendall *et al.*, 1997; Burton and Main, 2000), and cover a range of beliefs, attitudes, and expectations (Main and Burton, 2000):

- dysfunctional attitudes, beliefs, and expectations about pain and disability
- inappropriate attitudes, beliefs, and expectations about health care
- uncertainty, anxiety, fear-avoidance
- depression, distress, low mood, negative emotions
- passive or negative coping strategies (e.g. catastrophizing)
- lack of 'motivation' and readiness to change, failure to take personal responsibility for rehabilitation, awaiting a 'fix', lack of effort
- 'illness behaviour'

In principle, these psychological factors are also likely to act as obstacles to return to work, though the evidence is less robust than that for other obstacles (Waddell *et al.*, 2003). Perceptions and beliefs about one's health condition, about work, about the relationship between them, and about one's 'workability' (termed 'blue flags' (Main and Burton, 2000)) are likely to form more specific obstacles for return to work (as opposed to clinical recovery) (Kendall *et al.*, 1997; Burton and Main, 2000; Marhold *et al.*, 2002):

- attribution of health condition to work (whether to an 'accident/ injury' or to the physical or mental demands of work)
- beliefs that work is harmful, and that return to work will do further damage or be unsafe
- beliefs about being too sick/disabled to contemplate return to work
- beliefs that one cannot or should not become fully active or return to work until the health condition is completely cured
- expectation of increased pain or fatigue if work is resumed
- low expectations about return to work
- beliefs and expectations about (premature) retirement
- low job dissatisfaction
- lack of social support at work, relationships with co-workers and employer

Psychosocial aspects of work (such as job satisfaction and social support) are to some extent 'external', but personal perceptions and beliefs about these working conditions have an important and direct effect on individual behaviour. It has been shown empirically that multiple psychosocial aspects of work have a cumulative effect on sickness absence (Bartys *et al.*, 2003).

Environmental/social obstacles

Health professionals focus on personal, 'internal', biological, and psychological factors, but often neglect important 'external' social obstacles. Return to work is not simply a matter of health or health care; return to work depends on the workplace and the employer, so environmental and occupational obstacles may be as important as health-related obstacles. Return to work depends on organizational policy, process, and practice, which depend on employers' perceptions, beliefs, and attitudes (Howard, 2003). Examples of work-related and organizational perceptions acting as obstacles include (Feuerstein and Zastowny, 1999; Waddell *et al.*, 2003):

- inappropriate medical information and advice about work
- inappropriate sick certification practice

- employers' lack of understanding and assumption that back pain automatically means sickness absence
- belief by many employers that symptoms must be 'cured' before they can 'risk' permitting a return to work
- coworkers unhelpful attitudes and behaviours
- loss of contact and lack of communication between worker, employer, and health professionals

The individual and health care professionals may have no direct control over most of these occupational obstacles, but their effect may be powerfully influenced (for good or ill) by personal beliefs and the beliefs and behaviour of health professionals.

There are broader labour market and social security system obstacles, the pervasive nature and detrimental effects of which led to them being described as 'black flags' (Main and Burton, 2000); these can compromise delivery of effective interventions, but it is a mistake to think that means they are immutable – rather, they require a different kind of intervention. The person and health care clearly must operate within the existing 'system', but perceptions and behaviour by all the players can modulate the practice and outcomes of the system.

Bio-psycho-social interactions

For the sake of clarity, biological, psychological, and social obstacles have each been considered separately, which may give the impression that each of these dimensions is distinct, operates independently, and would require different interventions. In practice, there is no clear separation.

A strong theme underlying many of these obstacles is beliefs – by the person, the family, health professionals, coworkers, and employer. Beliefs may drive behaviour, and behaviour may drive beliefs, interactions between the players may mutually reinforce or conflict with each other. This can readily lead to uncertainty, which can afflict all the players.

Uncertainty may be a fundamental obstacle to recovery and return to work. People do not cope well when they are uncertain about what has gone wrong, about what the future holds, about what to do (or not to do), about whether to seek care (and from whom), about whether it is safe to return to work (and whether that can be sustained) (Indahl, 2003). Tackling uncertainty as a component of interventions for back pain is necessary but not sufficient, yet it may be fundamental to effective clinical and occupational management. Overcoming uncertainty, among all the players, may best be achieved through provision of suitable information and advice.

Tackling beliefs – getting the messages across

Education can target the beliefs that form obstacles to recovery/ return to work. Although education is a relatively weak intervention in itself, there is likely to be a knock-on effect, and there are numerous innovative studies looking at various delivery mechanisms in different settings. They all tend to demedicalize the experience of back pain, and address a common set of obstacles – disadvantageous beliefs that lead to uncertainty (Table 10.4). The interventions are focused on a small number of evidence-based messages about back pain that are equally appropriate to all the players: the spine is strong, rest is unhelpful, activity and exercise is good, work is beneficial, being gloomy is unhelpful, and doctors do not have the whole answer.

Symonds *et al.* developed a simple 'psychosocial' pamphlet focused on fear avoidance beliefs which, using the dichotomy between 'coper' and 'avoider', promoted the benefits of a positive outlook, the benefits of activity, and advised early return to work with back pain. This was compared with a traditional information pamphlet emphasizing good posture and correct lifting techniques (Symonds *et al.*, 1995). In a controlled trial, the pamphlets were broadcast to the entire workforce, and beliefs and absence measured over the following year. Compared with the controls, the workers at the factory receiving the psychosocial pamphlet showed a significant positive shift in beliefs and experienced a modest reduction in workloss.

The same basic set of messages has been extended and formulated as a more substantial booklet, *The Back Book* (Roland *et al.*, 1996; Roland *et al.*, 2002). This was developed initially as a clinical tool to accompany the UK guidelines

Table 10.4 Disadvantageous beliefs about back pain, disability and work – a few suitable targets

Beliefs about the inevitable consequences	Gets progressively worse Disability is likely Will stop you working You'll end up in a wheelchair
Beliefs about damage	There is permanent damage There is always a weakness
Fear avoidance beliefs	Physical activity or work will make it worse Physical activity or work caused it You can't work until the pain has gone Hurting means harming
Beliefs about treatment	Treatment is always needed Treatment will solve the problem No treatment before X-rays and scans

for the management of acute back pain in primary care (Royal College of General Practitioners, 1996). Written in simple language, the messages are presented in an uncompromising yet positive and helpful manner. The effectiveness of the booklet was tested in a controlled trial (Burton *et al.*, 1999). Primary care patients with back pain were randomly assigned to receive either *The Back Book* or a control booklet giving a traditional and virtually opposite set of messages; there were no other changes to usual treatment. Patients who received *The Back Book* had a significant reduction in disadvantageous beliefs, both short-term and at 12-months follow-up. Furthermore, those patients with high levels of fear avoidance beliefs at baseline experienced a significant reduction in disability at 12 months. This latter finding has also been reported in a study conducted in the US (George *et al.*, 2003). More recently, a study compared a single session of evidence-based information and advice with routine hands-on physiotherapy – both groups received *The Back Book*. It was concluded that routine physiotherapy seemed to be no more clinically effective than one session of assessment and advice, though the therapy group reported enhanced perceptions of benefit (Frost *et al.*, 2004).

The idea of using a lay person to lead a group education/ advice programme was studied in a randomized controlled trial in the US (Von Korff *et al.*, 1998). Delivered across four sessions, the programme used problem-solving techniques for the self-management of back pain, supplemented by a book and video giving similar messages to *The Back Book* but in much greater detail. The educational programme reduced worry and improved confidence, and also resulted in an improvement in self-rated disability. The same researchers carried out another trial of a somewhat similar programme delivered by a clinical psychologist over two sessions. The results broadly matched those from the lay-led programme but tended to occur faster (Moore *et al.*, 2000).

An award winning study in Australia used the same set of messages as the basis for a large multi-media public health campaign (Buchbinder *et al.*, 2001). Using television, print media, billboards, and the like, the campaign promoted an active approach to back pain management that included encouragement to stay at work. In addition, *The Back Book* was made freely available, and doctors were encouraged to foster the same approach. Outcomes were compared with those in a neighbouring state not exposed to the campaign. There was a significant positive shift in back beliefs during the campaign, which was sustained 3 years after the campaign finished (Buchbinder and Jolley, 2004). Importantly, there was an appreciable decline in the number workers' compensation claims, and a decline in the number of days compensated resulting in a 20 per cent reduction in cost-per-claim.

A similar, still unpublished, public health education campaign has been run in Scotland using the same messages (www.workingbacksscotland.com). As in Australia, there has been a sustained positive shift in back beliefs at the population level. Furthermore, there has been a change in the advice that doctors give to patients – with a substantial shift away from advising rest to advising an active approach. There are no data available yet on occupational outcomes.

In an Irish study, conducted in a social security setting, doctors were trained to use international evidence-based guidelines and consider workplace issues in the assessment of patients with back pain, with the intention of changing their practice in determination of workability (Leech, 2004). Also, claimants were invited for early assessment, and *The Back Book* was made freely available. Interestingly, on receipt of the invitation for assessment, 62 per cent of the claimants came off benefits and returned to work. During the study the assessors declared 64 per cent of those examined fit for work compared with around 20 per cent previously, and there were fewer appeals and fewer successful appeals. Although controlled using only retrospective comparison data, the study does suggest that it is possible, in this setting at least, to change both physician and claimant behaviour at an early stage in the disability process.

There is broad consensus on the importance of 'getting all the players onside' (Frank *et al.*, 1998), and this approach to providing an early supportive network has been studied in an occupational health environment (Burton *et al.*, 2005). Occupational health nurses were trained to implement a novel intervention protocol which involved very early contact with absent workers, an invitation to attend the occupational health unit for assessment, and steps to facilitate return to work. The protocol required the nurses to assess and address psychosocial issues using a cognitive behavioural approach, to maintain contact with the worker during absence, to liaise with the GP to minimize sick certification, and to liaise with the team leader to arrange temporary modified work if needed – therapy beyond attending the GP was specifically excluded. In a controlled trial, the results showed that the protocol, when followed, significantly reduced return to work time and also reduced further absence over the ensuing 12 months. Whilst certain psychosocial scores did improve following the intervention, it was not possible to identify which of the components of the package were most effective.

Conclusions

There is strong and consistent evidence that beliefs are important in back pain, as indeed they are in other common health problems; inappropriate beliefs can contribute to poor clinical outcomes and long-term incapacity

(Waddell *et al.*, 2003), and are major considerations for treatment and rehabilitation (Waddell and Burton, 2004). Whilst the beliefs of the patient are a major concern for healthcare, the beliefs and attitudes of all the players (health professionals, employers, and society) are inter-related and have an impact on what people do about their predicament when their back is hurting. Beliefs are only part of the back pain disability problem, but they can be tackled. The evidence suggests that appropriately focused educational interventions, across a range of environments, can shift beliefs and have a concomitant effect on clinical and vocational outcomes. Whilst the effect-size may be modest, in most instances it is similar to that found for medical interventions, and the overall benefits are likely to be cost effective. Further research is warranted to develop these innovative approaches, and to extend them to cover related issues such as sick certification and occupational health provision. It has been suggested that successful rehabilitation for common health problems (including back pain) requires a major cultural shift (Waddell and Burton, 2004); educational interventions targeting beliefs and attitudes can contribute to that process.

References

Balagué F, Dudler J and Nordin M (2003). Low back pain in children. *Lancet*, **361**, 1403–1404.

Bartys S, Burton K, Wright I, Mackay C, Watson P and Main C (2003). The influence of psychosocial risk factors on absence due to musculoskeletal disorders. In: PT McCabe, ed. *Contemporary ergonomics*, pp. 47–52. London: Taylor and Francis.

Buchbinder R and Jolley D (2004). Population based intervention to change back pain beliefs: three year follow up population survey. *British Medical Journal*, **328**, 321.

Buchbinder R, Jolley D and Wyatt M (2001). 2001 Volvo Award Winner in Clinical Studies: Effects of a media campaign on back pain beliefs and its potentional influence on management of low back pain in general practice. *Spine*, **26**, 2535–2542.

Burton AK and Main CJ (2000). Obstacles to recovery from work-related musculoskeletal disorders. In: W Karwowski, ed. *International encyclopedia of ergonomics and human factors*, pp. 1542–1544. London: Taylor and Francis.

Burton AK, Waddell G, Tillotson KM and Summerton N (1999). Information and advice to patients with back pain can have a positive effect: a randomized controlled trial of a novel educational booklet in primary care. *Spine*, **24**, 2484–2491.

Burton AK, McClune TD, Clarke RD and Main CJ (2004). Long-term follow-up of patients with low back pain attending for manipulative care: outcomes and predictors. *Manual Therapy*, **9**, 30–35.

Burton AK, Bartys S, Wright IA and Main CJ (2005). *Obstacles to recovery from musculoskeletal disorders in industry*. Research Report 323. London: HSE Books.

Chaudhary N, Longworth S and Sell PJ (2004). Management of mechanical low back pain – a survey of beliefs and attitudes in GPs from Leicester and Nottingham. *European Journal of General Practice*, **10**, 71–72.

Croft PR, Macfarlane GJ, Papageorgiou AC, Thomas E and Silman AJ (1998). Outcome of low back pain in general practice: a prospective study. *British Medical Journal*, **316**, 1356–1359.

Deyo RA (1998). Low back pain. *Scientific American*, **279**, 53.

Feuerstein M and Zastowny TR (1999). Occupational rehabilitation: multidisciplinary management of work-related musculoskeletal pain and disability. In: R Gatchel and DC Turk, ed. *Psychological approaches to pain management: a practitioner's handbook*, pp. 458–485. London: Guildford Press.

Frank J, Sinclair S, Hogg-Johnson S, Shannon H, Bombardier C, Beaton D and Cole D (1998). Preventing disability from work-related low-back pain. New evidence gives new hope – if we can just get all the players onside. *Canadian Medical Association Journal*, **158**, 1625–1631.

Frost H, Lamb SE, Doll HA, Carver PT and Stewart-Brown S (2004). Randomised controlled trial of physiotherapy compared with advice for low back pain. *British Medical Journal*, **329**(7468), 708.

George SZ, Fritz JM, Bialosky JE and Donald DA (2003). The effect of a fear-avoidance-based physical therapy intervention for patients with acute low back pain: results of a randomized controlled trial. *Spine*, **28**, 2551–2560.

Goubert L, Crombez G and De Bourdeaudhuij I (2004). Low back pain, disability and back pain myths in a community sample: prevalence and interrelationships. *European Journal of Pain*, **8**, 385–394.

Hadler NM (2001). Regional musculoskeletal 'injuries': a social construction. *Rheuma21st*. Available at: www.rheuma21st.com/archives/.

Hamonet C, Boulay C, Heiat A, Saraoui H, Boulongne D, Chignon JC, Wackenheim P, Macé Y, Rigal C and Staub H (2001). Les mots qui font mal. *Douleurs*, **2**, 29–33.

Howard M (2003). *An 'interactionist' perspective on barriers and bridges to work for disabled people*. IPPR, London. Available at: www.ippr.org/research/index.php?current=24&project=90.

Ihlebæk C and Eriksen HR (2003). Are the 'myths' of low back pain alive in the general Norwegian population? *Scandinavian Journal of Public Health*, **31**, 395–398.

Ihlebæk C and Eriksen HR (2004). The 'myths' of low back pain: Status quo in Norwegian general practitioners and physiotherapists. *Spine*, **29**, 1818–1822.

Indahl A (2003). *When the back acts up*. Rakkestad, Norway: Valdisholm forlag AS.

Jones MA, Stratton G, Reilly T and Unnithan VB (2004). A school-based survey of recurrent non-specific low-back pain prevalence and consequences in children. *Health Education Research*, **19**, 284–289.

Kendall NAS, Linton SJ and Main CJ (1997). *Guide to assessing psychosocial yellow flags in acute low back pain: Risk factors for long-term disability and work loss*. Wellington, NZ: Accident Rehabilitation and Compensation Insurance Corporation of New Zealand and the National Health Committee.

Leech C (2004). *Preventing chronic disability from low back pain – Renaissance Project*. Dublin: The Stationery Office, (Government Publications Office).

Main CJ and Burton AK (2000). Economic and occupational influences on pain and disability. In: CJ Main and CC Spanswick, ed. *Pain management. An interdisciplinary approach*, pp. 63–87. Edinburgh: Churchill Livingstone.

Main CJ and Spanswick CC (2000). *Pain management. An interdisciplinary approach.* Edinburgh: Churchill Livingstone.

Main CJ and Waddell G (2004). Beliefs about back pain. In: G Wadell, ed. *The back pain revolution*, pp. 221–240. Edinburgh: Churchill Livingstone.

Marhold C, Linton SJ and Melin L (2002). Identification of obstacles for chronic pain patients to return to work: Evaluation of a questionnaire. *Journal of Occupational Rehabilitation*, **12**, 65–75.

Klaber Moffett JA, Newbronner E, Waddell G, Croucher K and Spear S (2000). Public perceptions about low back pain and its management: a gap between expectations and reality? *Health Expectations*, **3**, 161–168.

Moon SD (1996). A psychosocial view of cumulative trauma disorders: implications for occupational health and prevention. In: SD Moon and SL Sauter, ed. *Beyond biomechanics: psychosocial aspects of musculoskeletal disorders in office work*, pp. 109–144. London: Taylor and Francis.

Moore JE, Von Korff M, Cherkin D, Saunders K and Lorig K (2000). A randomized trial of a cognitive-behavioral program for enhancing back pain self care in a primary care setting. *Pain*, **88**, 145–154.

Page LA and Wessely S (2003). Medically unexplained symptoms: exacerbating factors in the doctor-patient encounter. *Journal of the Royal Society of Medicine*, **96**, 223–227.

Pincus T and Morley S (2002). Cognitive appraisal. In: SJ Linton, ed. *New avenues for the prevention of chronic musculoskeletal pain and disability. Pain research and clinical management*, vol. 12, pp. 123–141. Amsterdam: Elsevier.

Roland M, Waddell G, Klaber Moffett J, Burton K and Main C (2002). *The back book.* London: The Stationery Office (www.tso.co.uk).

Roland M, Waddell G, Klaber-Moffett J, Burton K, Main C and Cantrell T (1996). *The back book.* London: The Stationery Office (www.tso.co.uk).

Royal College of General Practitioners (1996). *Clinical guidelines for the management of acute low back pain.* London: Royal College of General Practitioners.

Royal College of General Practitioners (1999). *Clinical guidelines for the management of acute low back pain.* London: Royal College of General Practitioners (www.rcgp.org.uk).

Symonds TL, Burton AK, Tillotson KM and Main CJ (1995). Absence resulting from low back trouble can be reduced by psychosocial intervention at the work place. *Spine*, **20**, 2738–2745.

Symonds TL, Burton AK, Tillotson KM and Main CJ (1996). Do attitudes and beliefs influence work loss due to low back trouble? *Occupational Medicine*, **46**, 25–32.

Ursin H (1997). Sensitization, somatisation, and subjective health complaints: a review. *International Journal of Behavioral Medicine*, **4**, 427–436.

Von Korff M and Moore JC (2001). Stepped care for back pain: activating approaches for primary care. *Annals of Internal Medicine*, **134**, 911–917.

Von Korff M, Moore JE, Lorig K, Cherkin DC, Saunders K, Gonzalez VM, Laurent D, Rutter C and Comite F (1998). A randomized trial of a lay person-led self-management group intervention for back pain patients in primary care. *Spine*, **23**, 2608–2615.

Waddell G (2004). *The back pain revolution.* Edinburgh: Churchill Livingstone.

Waddell G and Burton AK (2004). *Concepts of rehabilitation for the management of common health problems.* London: The Stationery Office.

Waddell G, Burton AK and Main CJ (2003). *Screening to identify people at risk of long-term incapacity for work.* London: Royal Society of Medicine Press.

Waxman R, Tennant A and Helliwell P (1998). Community survey of factors associated with consultation for low back pain. *British Medical Journal,* **317**, 1564–1567.

Chapter 11

Managing disability by public policy initiatives

Rachelle Buchbinder

Introduction

Preventive health initiatives deliver a range of health messages to the public designed to influence population attitudes and beliefs and lead to a change in health risk behaviours. Wide dissemination of health information, such as through the mass media, plays a potentially vital role in the success of these initiatives. The media has been shown to be a leading source of information about important health issues (Redman *et al.*, 1990). It is also a means for reaching larger numbers of people at less expense than that associated with face-to-face services. As well as disseminating information to the general population, the popular press has also been shown to amplify the transmission of medical information to the scientific community (Phillips *et al.*, 1991).

The World Health Organization's Ottawa Charter for Health Promotion has identified media advocacy as an established health promotion strategy (Grilli *et al.*, 2002). The media has been used to influence behaviour of patients and health professionals, and promote effective and efficient use of health services (Grilli *et al.*, 2002). For example it has been used to alter a wide variety of health-related behaviours such as smoking (Sly *et al.*, 2001), sunlight exposure (Hill *et al.*, 1993), and physical activity (Owen *et al.*, 1995). It has also been used to promote use of health-care interventions such as preventive asthma therapy, cancer and HIV screening, immunization programmes, and emergency services for suspected myocardial infarction (Grilli *et al.*, 2002).

Public policy initiatives that aim to influence population beliefs have been particularly successful in Australia in altering health-related behaviours such as smoking (Pierce *et al.*, 1990) and sunlight exposure (Hill *et al.*, 1993). Widespread primary prevention public health campaigns relating to sunlight exposure have been operating in Australia for 20 years (Marks, 1999). The effect of these programmes has been to create a very large shift in knowledge, attitudes, and beliefs about sunlight exposure and suntans, along with major shifts in behaviour. Suntans have become less popular, sunlight exposure has been reduced, and this has been accompanied by a significant reduction in sunburn and skin cancer incidence and mortality rates (Marks, 1999).

An advantage of public policy health initiatives over more targeted initiatives is their ability to reach groups who are difficult to access through traditional medical delivery (Redman *et al.*, 1990). Public policy initiatives have the potential to modify the knowledge or attitudes of a large proportion of the community simultaneously, thereby providing social support for behavioural change (Redman *et al.*, 1990). The presence of social support may help to maintain behavioural change over time.

In 1997, the Victorian WorkCover Authority, the manager of the Australian state of Victoria's workers' compensation system, identified the need to tackle the rising costs of workers' compensation costs for back pain claims. The workers' compensation system had paid out $A385 million dollars for back pain claims in the state of Victoria during the 1996/1997 12-month financial period, and this figure had tripled over a decade (Victorian WorkCover Authority, 1996). It was recognized that the traditional biomedical approach to back pain management was contributing to the escalating costs and that strategies to change clinical practice in line with the best available evidence were required.

A health professional advisory committee was set up, whose main task was to identify a limited number of key messages about back pain that would have the support of all key stakeholders. However, it was recognized by the Director of Public Affairs of the Victorian WorkCover Authority and others that targeting health care providers alone would have limited impact upon changing clinical practice, and a novel approach that would spread the message to the general public, employers, workers, and patients was required. It was well accepted that Australia had a history of successful public health campaigns, and, at the same time, data was being published suggesting that improved outcomes from back pain could be achieved by provision of simple information and advice addressing psychosocial factors (Symonds *et al.*, 1995).

On this basis, the Victorian WorkCover Authority embarked upon a groundbreaking approach to the prevention and management of disability from low back pain. A 3-year population-based, mass media campaign entitled 'Back Pain: Don't Take It Lying Down', aimed to reduce back-pain-related disability by challenging the traditional attitudes towards back problems and shifting beliefs in line with modern thinking. The campaign resulted in significant improvements in both community and doctors' beliefs about back pain and this was accompanied by a decline in the number of back claims and medical payments over the duration of the campaign (Buchbinder *et al.*, 2001a).

Furthermore, a recent follow-up survey has shown that 3 years after cessation of the campaign, there are still significant, sustained improvements in community beliefs about back pain (Buchbinder and Jolley, 2004).

This chapter will describe the rationale for a public health policy approach to back pain disability, details of the campaign itself, and results of an independent evaluation of its outcome. We will show that this data provides a compelling evidence-based case for managing other public health issues that are strongly influenced by attitudes and beliefs, by similar public policy initiatives.

Rationale for a public health policy approach to back pain disability

Extent of the problem

Based upon population-based surveys, the lifetime prevalence of back pain is reported to be 60 to 80 per cent, with a point prevalence of 15 to 30 per cent and a 1-year prevalence of 50 per cent (Nachemson et al., 2000). Back pain is the second most common symptom leading to general practitioner consultation after upper respiratory complaints (Cypress, 1983; Bridges-Webb et al., 1992; Hart et al., 1995). It is the most common cause of activity limitation in adults less than 45 years and the fourth most common in those aged 45 to 64 years (Andersson, 1997). Most episodes of acute low back pain improve, although longitudinal studies suggest that back pain is often persistent and typically a recurrent condition (von Korff, 1994; Cherkin et al., 1996; Croft et al., 1998; van den Hoogen et al., 1998; Schiottz-Christensen et al., 1999). Nevertheless, the majority of people with acute back pain are able to resume normal function and return to work quickly whether the pain has fully resolved or not (von Korff, 1994; van den Hoogen et al., 1998; Schiottz-Christensen et al., 1999).

Despite the good prognosis of acute low back pain and increasing scientific evidence for simple conservative management (van Tulder et al., 1997; Waddell et al., 1997), back-pain-related disability is becoming an increasing public health concern in developed countries worldwide. This is highlighted by the fact that back pain is one of the major issues being addressed in the Bone and Joint Decade of 2000–2010 (Brooks and Hart, 2000). For example, in Australia, back problems are the leading specific musculoskeletal cause of health-system expenditure with an estimated total cost of $A700 million dollars in 1993–1994 (Mathers and Penn, 1999) and these costs are rising. While back pain accounts for about one-third of all workers' compensation lost-time claims, it accounts for 40 per cent of all long-term claims and almost 50 per cent of the total costs.

Back pain also places a significant socioeconomic burden upon the individual. Estimates of the costing for workers' compensation suggest that the costs for employers have been at least matched by similar amounts for the individual and the community (Industry Commission Report, 1995). Chronic back pain may lead to isolation, depression, lengthy absences from work, and unemployment in the long-term (Hendler, 1984). Back-pain-related disability is also frequently associated with family disruption, loss of self-esteem and quality of life (Philips and Jahanshahi, 1986; Zarkowska and Philips, 1986).

Patient attitudes and beliefs are strongly linked to disability

Since the mid-1980s patients' attitudes and beliefs, particularly fear-avoidance beliefs, pain-coping strategies, and illness behaviours, have been increasingly recognized to be important predictors of outcome (Lethem *et al.*, 1983; Waddell, 1987; Waddell *et al.*, 1993; Symonds *et al.*, 1996). They are strongly associated with the shift from acute to chronic back pain disability and are more influential than biomedical or biomechanical factors (Burton *et al.*, 1995; Klenerman *et al.*, 1995; Linton, 2000).

The fear-avoidance model has been used to explain why a small minority of people with low back pain develop chronic problems while the majority recover spontaneously, on the basis of individual differences in response to painful stimuli that can be seen in terms of a continuum of fear of pain (Klenerman *et al.*, 1995). On the one hand, there are 'confronters' who have minimal fear of pain and are able to gradually increase their exposure to painful activities and rehabilitate themselves. 'Avoiders' on the other hand, have a strong fear of pain leading them to avoid activities that may exacerbate their pain, which leads to other somatic consequences such as loss of mobility and muscular strength, which in turn reinforces avoidance behaviour and the sick role (Klenerman *et al.*, 1995). The predictive value of this explanatory model has been shown for individuals with both acute and chronic low back pain, signifying the importance of psychosocial factors in both the assessment and management of low back pain (Waddell *et al.*, 1993; Klenerman *et al.*, 1995).

Patients' concerns about the seriousness of their condition, the explanatory models they construct to understand their symptoms, and their general views and expectations also influence the development of chronic disability (Kravitz *et al.*, 1997).

Health care provider beliefs linked to treatment approaches

Management of back pain based upon the biomedical model is increasingly accepted as playing an important role in back disability (Waddell, 1987; Loeser and Sullivan, 1995). Individual clinical treatments have had limited impact upon long-term outcomes for back pain (Deyo, 1996a; van der Weide et al., 1997). There is only modest evidence that treatment significantly helps symptoms (van Tulder et al., 1997), and a substantial amount of evidence about the adverse effects of rest, surgery, medication, and focusing on the problem itself (Indahl et al., 1995; Malmivaara et al., 1995; Deyo, 1996a).

Despite increasing evidence that positive advice to stay active and continue or resume ordinary activities is more efficacious than rest (Waddell et al., 1997) and early investigation and specialist referral are unwarranted in the majority of cases (Deyo and Phillips, 1996), surveys of physicians continue to demonstrate only partial adoption of these management strategies (Cherkin et al., 1995; Little et al., 1996). This, in part, may reflect physicians' knowledge and beliefs (Cherkin et al., 1995). Surveys of physicians and other health care providers, including physiotherapists and chiropractors, have repeatedly demonstrated that treatment approaches vary according to the health care provider's beliefs about back pain causation (Cherkin et al., 1988; Battie et al., 1994; Rainville et al., 2000; Ostelo et al., 2003). A recent study was able to discriminate between physiotherapists with either a biomedical or biopsychosocial treatment orientation based upon their opinion towards various aspects of management of chronic low back pain (Ostelo et al., 2003).

Disability associated with low back pain viewed within a social context

Development of disability will also be influenced by societal factors such as current community views, political agendas of governing powers, and the existing legislation regarding sickness absence and compensation. While management of low back pain will be shaped by the health-care provider's knowledge, beliefs, and training, it may also be influenced by societal factors. Social influences have been shown to play a more important role than scientific influences in shaping the behaviour and medical decisions of physicians (Dixon, 1990). The patient's presentation of their symptoms, and their knowledge, beliefs, and expectations from the encounter, may all influence management (Owen et al., 1990; Freeborn et al., 1997; Little et al., 1998; Chew-Graham and May, 1999). Patient satisfaction, provision of reassurance, relationship to work, and maintenance of the doctor–patient relationship have all been shown to be important psychosocial determinants of physicians' behaviour when managing back pain.

Efforts by employers to accommodate the low back pain sufferer at work have also been shown to be important in reducing the duration of disability due to back pain (Loisel et al., 1997; Rossignol et al., 2000). Appropriate modification of work duties, enabling either no lost time or early return to work, has been shown to reduce both the duration of back claims and the incidence of new back claims (Frank *et al.*, 1998). Newer studies of guideline-based approaches to back pain in the workplace suggest that co-ordinated, workplace-linked care systems can achieve a reduction of 50 per cent in time lost due to back pain at no extra cost and in some settings with significant savings (Frank *et al.*, 1998).

Satisfaction with medical care linked to provision of information

The evidence suggests patients' satisfaction with care to be most highly correlated with provision of information (Deyo and Diehl, 1986; von Korff *et al.*, 1994; Carey *et al.*, 1995; Skelton *et al.*, 1996). In a qualitative review of back pain management, Skelton *et al.* found that only 22 of 55 patients reported satisfaction with levels of primary care (Skelton *et al.*, 1996). The main reported issues of concern were communication and thoroughness and 21 patients reported dissatisfaction with the practitioners' ability to provide an adequate explanation of the problem. von Korff *et al.* found that patient satisfaction with primary care management was positively correlated with emphasis on provision of information and advice on self-management of back pain, versus the traditional approach of prescribing analgesics and bed rest (von Korff *et al.*, 1994). Carey *et al.* reviewed consecutive patients attending medical and chiropractic practices and found that less than 50 per cent of patients were satisfied with the information provided, the treatment of their back problem, and the overall result of treatment (Carey *et al.*, 1995). Deyo *et al.* found patients with back pain expressed a need for more and better-quality information about their condition (Deyo and Diehl, 1986). Unmet needs were also associated with poorer compliance and a desire for more investigation or evaluation. These studies all suggest that primary care physicians and others may lack knowledge, and/or skills, and/or confidence in imparting information about back pain.

Improved outcome associated with provision of information and advice addressing psychosocial factors

A variety of studies have now shown that an informative approach designed to promote a positive approach to low back pain and address fear-avoidance beliefs and poor coping strategies improves outcomes (Roland and Dixon, 1989; Symonds *et al.*, 1995; Burton *et al.*, 1999). Roland *et al.* found than an educational pamphlet about low back trouble reduced consultation rates in a primary care clinic (Roland and Dixon, 1989). Provision of positive messages designed to improve back beliefs and reduce fear has also been shown to reduce self-reported disability in those presenting with low back pain in general practice (Burton *et al.*, 1999). In an industrial setting, Symonds *et al.* demonstrated that distribution of an educational psychosocial pamphlet designed to foster positive beliefs and attitudes successfully reduced absenteeism (Symonds *et al.*, 1995). They observed that the reduction in extended work absence occurred in those with and without pre-existing back complaints (Symonds *et al.*, 1995). The benefits of these approaches may far outweigh those derived from specific traditional treatments (Indahl *et al.*, 1995).

Deyo *et al.* also showed that an educational intervention designed to modify patient expectation can reduce inappropriate imaging and costs, without compromising symptom resolution, functional improvement, satisfaction, or detection of serious pathology (Deyo *et al.*, 1987).

Translating research findings into clinical practice

Attempts to implement research findings into practice and change physicians' behaviour have met with limited success (Bero *et al.*, 1998; Wensig *et al.*, 1998). While some studies have shown that general practitioners manage back pain appropriately (Maetzel *et al.*, 2000), others have found that traditional approaches, such as bed rest and early imaging and physiotherapy referral, continue to prevail (Schroth *et al.*, 1992; Cherkin *et al.*, 1995; Elam *et al.*, 1995; Carey and Garrett, 1996; Little *et al.*, 1996; Freeborn *et al.*, 1997).

Passive dissemination of information is generally unsuccessful in influencing behaviour in general practice (Bero *et al.*, 1998), whereas combinations of information transfer, learning through social influence or management support, as well as reminders or feedback seem to be effective (Wensig *et al.*, 1998). A co-ordinated system of care, which accommodates physician and patient preferences, meets patient needs for adequate explanation and participation in decision making, and establishes an ongoing relationship with a caring provider, has been shown to effect behaviour change and improve outcomes (Rossignol *et al.*, 2000).

Changing physician behaviour is very complex – it involves enhancing know-ledge, changing attitudes and beliefs, providing necessary skills and resources, and providing support and feedback (van Tulder *et al.*, 2002). There are many potential sources of variation in managing an individual presenting with acute low back pain. Modifying one source of variation without concomitantly considering the effect (or lack of effect) on other factors may lead to failure to effect a change in outcome. For example educational updates and clinical guide-lines about back pain may improve physician knowledge but may not effect a change in behaviour (and final outcome) if patient expectation or the doctor's beliefs about patient expectation or environmental influences remain the same. Management of low back pain commonly involves other physicians, including orthopaedic surgeons, rheumatologists, rehabilitation physicians, and radiologists, and other health professionals including physiotherapists and chiropractors, yet most research on changing management has been directed towards primary care. It is not known whether the issues regarding changing behaviour will be equally applicable to other groups.

Shifting societal views about back pain

While the biopsychosocial model of back pain proposed by Waddell (Waddell, 1987) and others in the mid-1980s is now well accepted among back pain experts, there is abundant evidence that this fundamental shift from the traditional medical model of back pain has yet to be universally adopted. Recent qualitative studies have highlighted the current disparity between the low back pain patient's physical model of pain causation and the doctors' psychosocial model (Chew-Graham and May, 1999). Doctors feel ill-equipped to challenge the patient's model without damaging the doctor–patient relationship and, in any case, may be unable to influence the social factors that shape the patient's presentation (Chew-Graham and May, 1997). Patients' views and beliefs about the cause and prognosis of their back pain and about the most effective treatments may not correspond to the care proposed by the evidence (van Tulder *et al*, 1997). With increasing emphasis on patient participation and shared decision making, patients' views and beliefs may influence the process and outcome of consultations. As previously suggested by Deyo, it may be that the public as well as the medical profession need to be re-educated (Deyo, 1996b). If re-education can change population attitudes and beliefs and give rise to a concomitant alteration in patient expectation and physician behaviour, this may be effective in stemming or reversing the rising epidemic of low back pain disability (Buchbinder *et al.*, 2001a).

The Victorian WorkCover Authority back pain campaign

The Victorian WorkCover Authority back pain campaign was based upon the messages delineated in *The Back Book*, an evidence-based patient educational booklet produced in the UK by a multidisciplinary team of authors (Roland *et al.*, 1996). The messages were simple and in line with current evidence: back pain is not a serious medical problem; disability can be improved and even prevented by positive attitudes; treatment should consist of continuing to perform usual activities, not resting for prolonged periods, exercising, and remaining at work (Burton *et al.*, 1999). It counselled individuals with low back pain, their doctors, and employers to avoid excessive medicalization of the problem, unnecessary diagnostic testing and treatment. It tackled fear-avoidance beliefs and promoted gradual exposure to painful activities, emphasizing that it was unlikely to be harmful. To ensure that the campaign did not discourage patients with serious pathology from seeking early medical assessment, advertisements highlighting 'red flag' symptoms were also shown.

The campaign included electronic, print, and outdoor media and targeted both the community and treating doctors. The major medium of the campaign was television commercials that were aired in prime time slots commencing in September 1997. The intensity of the campaign varied, with a concentrated campaign for 3 months initially followed by a low-key maintenance campaign until September 1998. A further 3-month concentrated television campaign commenced in September 1999 followed by a low-key maintenance campaign until February 2000.

The commercials included recognized international and national medical experts in orthopaedic surgery, rehabilitation, rheumatology, general practice, physiotherapy, chiropractic therapy, and sports and occupational medicine. There were also advertisements by well known sporting and local television personalities characters who had successfully managed their own back pain. All advertisements concluded with endorsements by the relevant national or state professional medical bodies. Virtually every professional body with a stake in back pain in Australia supported the campaign and had input into the wording and content of the advertisements.

Radio, billboard advertisements, posters, seminars, visits by personalities to workplaces, publicity articles, and publications supported the television campaign. *The Back Book* was sent to all treating practitioners in Victoria to be given to patients suffering from back pain, and in the latter stages of the campaign to insurers to be passed on to claimants. Guidelines for the management of employees with compensable low back pain, developed over a 3-year period with consultation from a wide variety of treating practitioners (Victorian WorkCover Authority, 1996), were also introduced simultaneously.

Evaluation of the impact of the Victorian WorkCover Authority mass media back campaign

We undertook an independent three-part evaluation of the campaign to determine the impact of the campaign upon population beliefs about back pain, the knowledge and attitudes of Victorian general practitioners as well as its effect on workers' compensation back claims over time (Buchbinder *et al.*, 2001a; 2001b).

Population beliefs

The effect of the campaign on population beliefs was measured by conducting telephone surveys of three separate cross-sectional, random samples of the employed population prior to the campaign and 2 and 2.5 years after campaign onset. The telephone surveys were conducted in Victoria and New South Wales, an adjacent state where we knew no public health campaign for back pain was to take place for the duration of our study. Both states have similar demographic characteristics and worker's compensation systems.

There were 4730 surveys completed, with equal numbers in each state, and a ratio of 2 : 1 : 1 across the three time periods. Demographic characteristics and previous experience of back pain were similar at each time point both within and between states. At baseline about half of the respondents in both states had been aware of back pain advertising in the previous year (Vic 47.1 per cent, NSW 51.5 per cent). While this did not change over time in NSW (48.5 per cent and 48.0 per cent for Survey 2 and 3 respectively), there was a significant increase in awareness of back pain advertising in Victoria (73.9 and 85.5 per cent for Survey 2 and 3 respectively; $p < 0.001$). This was accompanied by a self-reported change in beliefs about back pain as a consequence of advertising (23.1, 38.8 and 48.0 per cent at Surveys 1–3 respectively; $p < 0.001$) (Buchbinder et al., 2001a).

The primary measure of beliefs about back pain was the Back Beliefs Questionnaire which is a self-administered questionnaire designed to measure beliefs about the inevitable consequences of future life with low back trouble (Symonds et al., 1995). A higher score indicates a more positive belief about low back trouble, suggesting better ability to cope with low back pain. At baseline, mean Back Beliefs Questionnaire scores were similar in both states (Table 11.1). There were significant improvements in mean scores in Victoria between successive surveys, whereas mean scores were unchanged in NSW across time (Buchbinder et al., 2001a).

At baseline the distribution of Back Belief Questionnaire scores within the population was almost identical in both states. This is illustrated in a quantile–quantile plot as shown in Fig. 11.1 (plot on left). The quantiles of the Victorian distribution of scores are shown on the horizontal axis interpolated against the quantiles of the NSW distribution of scores shown on the vertical axis. A quantile–quantile plot displays exact quantiles of one distribution against interpolated quantiles of a comparison set. Identical distributions (as in this case) are characterized by points that lie mostly on a 45° line from lower left to upper right.

Quantile–quantile plots are particularly useful in assessing the homogeneity or uniformity in location shift between two distributions; points that lie on a

Table 11.1 Back Beliefs Questionnaire; mean scores and difference in mean score from Survey 1 by state (Victoria, New South Wales) and survey (1, August 1997; 2, August 1999; 3, February 2000; 4, December 2002)

State	Survey	n	Mean score (95% CI)	Difference in mean score from Survey 1 (95% CI)	P-value
Victoria	1	1185	26.5 (26.1–26.8)		
	2	590	28.4 (27.9–28.8)	1.9 (1.3 to 2.5)	<0.001
	3	592	29.7 (29.2–30.3)	3.2 (2.6 to 3.9)	<0.001
	4	900	28.8 (28.4–29.2)	2.3 (1.8 to 2.8)	<0.001
NSW	1	1185	26.3 (25.9–26.6)		
	2	590	26.2 (25.7–26.7)	−0.04 (−0.7 to 0.6)	0.9
	3	588	26.3 (25.7–26.8)	0.02 (−0.6 to 0.7)	1.0
	4	600	26.1 (25.5–26.6)	0.02 (−0.8 to 0.4)	0.6

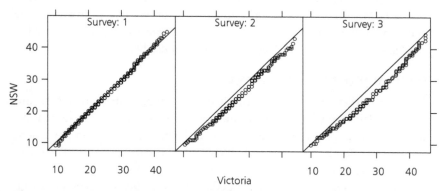

Fig. 11.1 Quantile–quantile plots of Back Beliefs Questionnaire for Victoria compared to New South Wales according to Survey (1 – August 1997; 2 – August 1999; 3 – February 2000).

straight line parallel to the leading diagonal are strong evidence of homogeneity in location shift between two distributions. At Survey 2 (middle plot) the points are uniformly shifted to the right of the 45° line, indicating that Back Beliefs Questionnaire scores are generally higher in Victoria compared with NSW across the range of scores. At Survey 3 (plot on right) the points are generally shifted further to the right of the 45° line with more shift in the middle Back Beliefs Questionnaire score range indicating greater differences in distribution of scores in the mid-range.

Statistically significant improvements in mean Back Beliefs Questionnaire scores in Victoria were seen between successive surveys irrespective of age, sex, education level, employment status, type of work (manual or not), income, previous back pain experience, whether respondents reported awareness of back pain advertising or not, and irrespective of whether attitudes were reported to have changed as a result of seeing an advertising campaign (Buchbinder *et al.*, 2001a; 2001b).

A modified Fear Avoidance Beliefs Questionnaire was also administered to respondents who reported back pain in the past year. This instrument measures an individual's beliefs about physical or work activity being the cause of their trouble, and their fears about the dangers of such activities when they have an episode of low back trouble (Waddell *et al.*, 1993). It has two subscales: physical activity and work. For both components, a lower score indicates less fear-avoidance beliefs. Significant improvements in mean fear avoidance beliefs about physical activity were observed in Victoria between successive surveys with a mean improvement of -1.5 and -2.4 between baseline and Surveys 2 and 3 respectively, with no changes observed in NSW (Table 11.2). Fear avoidance beliefs about work did not change in either state between baseline and Survey 2 but changed in both states between baseline and Survey 3 ($p = 0.02$ in NSW) (Buchbinder *et al.*, 2001b).

General practitioner surveys

A mailed survey of a random sample of general practitioners before and 2.5 years after campaign commencement was also performed. The design was similar to the population surveys in that a non-randomized, non-equivalent before–after design was used with NSW acting as control group. The questionnaire was modified from a questionnaire developed in Ontario, Canada (Bombardier *et al.*, 1995) and included a set of questions aimed at eliciting knowledge about: the management of acute low back pain; attitudes towards these patients; and attitudes towards management guidelines. The questions were phrased as statements and responses were on a five-point Likert scale that varied from 'strongly agree' to 'strongly disagree'. Respondents' likely approach to management of acute and subacute low back pain was also elicited, based upon presentation of two hypothetical scenarios.

There were 2556 surveys completed. As for the population surveys, the number of doctors who were aware of a back pain media campaign rose significantly in Victoria between successive surveys (from 15.5 per cent at Survey 1 to 89.3 per cent at Survey 2; $p < 0.001$). This was accompanied by a rise from 3.3 per cent to 31.9 per cent of doctors who reported that the campaign had changed their beliefs about back pain ($p < 0.001$) (Buchbinder *et al.*, 2001a).

Table 11.2 Fear Avoidance Beliefs Questionnaire; mean scores and difference in mean score from Survey 1 by state (Victoria, New South Wales) and survey (1, August 1997; 2, August 1999; 3, February 2000)

State	Survey	n	Mean score (95% CI)	Difference in mean score from Survey 1 (95% CI)	P-value
Fear avoidance beliefs about physical activity					
Victoria	1	640	14.0 (13.6–14.4)		
	2	343	12.5 (11.9–13.1)	−1.5 (−2.2 to −0.8)	0.000
	3	307	11.6 (11.0–12.2)	−2.4 (−3.1 to −1.6)	0.000
NSW	1	645	13.3 (12.9–13.8)		
	2	317	13.6 (13.1–14.2)	0.3 (−0.4 to 1.0)	0.411
	3	274	12.7 (12.0–13.5)	−0.6 (−1.4 to 0.2)	0.165
Fear avoidance beliefs about work (modified)					
Victoria	1	640	13.5 (12.7–14.2)		
	2	343	14.5 (13.5–15.5)	1.1 (−0.2 to 2.3)	0.105
	3	307	12.5 (11.3–13.6)	−1.0 (−2.3 to 0.3)	0.146
NSW	1	645	13.7 (12.9–14.4)		
	2	317	13.6 (12.5–14.6)	−0.1 (−1.4 to 1.2)	0.891
	3	274	12.1 (11.0–13.2)	−1.6 (−2.9 to −0.2)	0.020

The results are shown in Tables 11.3 and 11.4 and, in general, support the hypothesis that the media campaign in Victoria changed physician beliefs and attitudes towards low back pain, and stated likely management of acute and subacute low back pain. For example, over time, Victorian doctors were 3.6 (2.4–5.6) times as likely to know that patients with low back pain need not wait to be almost pain free to return to work (Table 11.3). They were also 2.9 (1.6–5.2) times as likely to know that patients with acute low back pain should not be prescribed complete bed rest until the pain goes away and 1.6 (1.2–2.3) times as likely to know that X-rays of the lumbar spine are not useful in the work up of acute low back pain. Victorian doctors also indicated that they would be less likely to order tests for low back pain either because patients expect them to (OR = 1.6; 95 per cent CI 1.1–2.3) or to conform with the normal practice patterns of their peer group (OR = 1.5; 95 per cent CI 1.1–2.0) (Buchbinder et al., 2001a).

Over time, Victorian doctors were 2.51 times as likely not to order tests for acute low back pain and 0.40 times as likely to order lumbosacral X-rays (Table 11.4). They were also 0.48 times as likely to prescribe bed rest and

Table 11.3 Responses to statements about back pain according to state (Victoria, New South Wales) and survey (1, August 1997; 2, February 2000) and ratio of odds ratios for change between survey, Victoria versus NSW

Statement		Response (%) State				Interaction odds ratios (95% CI)[1]	P-value
		Victoria Survey wave (Number of respondents)		NSW			
		1 (691)	2 (562)	1 (791)	2 (512)		
Knowledge							
Patients with LBP should not return to work until they are almost pain free	Correct response[2] Disagree	68.5	90.2	77.8	80.2	3.6 (2.4–5.6)	0.000
Patients with acute LBP should be prescribed complete bed rest until pain goes away	Disagree	77.1	96.0	80.9	91.3	2.9 (1.6–5.2)	0.000
X-rays of the lumbar spine are useful in the work up of acute (<1 month) LBP	Disagree	60.4	72.3	64.2	65.4	1.6 (1.2–2.3)	0.004
Encouragement of physical activity is important in the recovery of LBP	Agree	91.0	98.7	92.0	97.6	2.2 (0.8–6.0)	0.131
Back education programs aimed at educating workers in safe lifting techniques are effective in reducing recurrences of LBP	Uncertain Disagree	4.3	3.5	6.6	3.4	1.6 (0.7–3.6)	0.267

In patients with LBP and neurological findings in the long term there is no difference between surgical and medical management (excluding cauda equina)	Agree	24.9	27.5	22.1	28.1	0.8 (0.6–1.2)	0.307
Interventions by doctors and other providers in the health care system have very little positive impact on the natural history of acute LBP	Agree	32.1	33.9	26.0	34.2	0.7 (0.5–1.0)	0.077
The following treatment modalities are effective in managing most acute LBP:							
NSAIDS	Agree	83.2	87.0	86.4	87.5	1.2 (0.8–1.9)	0.393
Traction	Disagree	45.3	52.1	44.3	54.2	0.9 (0.6–1.2)	0.443
TENS	Disagree	24.3	28.1	27.1	28.8	0.9 (0.8–1.4)	0.418
Manipulation	Uncertain	21.3	20.9	20.4	26.9	0.7 (0.5–1.0)	0.066
Acupuncture	Disagree	18.0	19.3	20.2	21.0	1.0 (0.7–1.6)	0.848
Attitudes							
I am likely to order X-rays for LBP because patients so often expect me to do so	Positive response Disagree	69.0	79.2	72.1	73.1	1.6 (1.1–2.3)	0.010
Many of the investigations for my patients with LBP are ordered to conform with the normal practice patterns of my peer group	Disagree	52.7	60.1	57.0	55.1	1.5 (1.1–2.0)	0.020

Table 11.3 (Continued)

Statement		Response (%) State				Interaction odds ratios (95% CI)[1]	P-value
		Victoria Survey wave (Number of respondents)		NSW			
		1 (691)	2 (562)	1 (791)	2 (512)		
There is nothing physically wrong with many patients with chronic back pain	Disagree	64.8	67.5	67.5	63.5	1.3 (0.9–1.9)	0.277
I often have negative feelings about treating people who have LBP	Disagree	58.5	64.4	54.9	57.3	1.2 (0.8–1.6)	0.131
Well motivated patients are unlikely to have long-term problems with low back pain	Agree	60.2	69.7	58.9	66.7	1.1 (0.8–1.5)	0.621
I have no difficulty in assessing the motivation of my LBP patients	Agree	33.1	37.0	30.1	38.7	0.8 (0.6–1.1)	0.215
Guidelines							
Practice guidelines are useful to help doctors in the management of medical conditions	Agree	71.1	83.6	72.8	82.1	1.2 (0.8–1.8)	0.534
I would find practice guidelines helpful in the management of low back pain	Agree	69.9	78.8	71.2	77.9	1.1 (0.8–1.6)	0.342

[1] Interaction between State of practice and survey wave; OR >1 implies change over time differs between States

[2] Correct response based upon authors' interpretation of the latest synthesis of the evidence

Table 11.4 Responses to scenarios by state and survey wave and ratio of odds ratios for change between survey waves, Victoria versus NSW

Scenario	Response (%) State				Ratio of odds ratio[1] Vic: NSW (95% CI)
	Victoria Survey (Number of completed surveys)		New South Wales		
	1 (691)	2 (562)	1 (791)	2 (512)	
Stated management of acute low back pain					
Would not order tests	60.5	74.2	68.3	61.7	2.51 (1.79–3.51)
Would order lumbosacral X-rays	32.0	19.8	24.0	29.5	0.40 (0.28–0.57)
Special imaging (CT, MRI, myelogram)	2.3	2.1	1.6	3.7	0.40 (0.14–1.13)
Would prescribe bed rest	39.9	14.6	34.3	21.9	0.48 (0.33–0.70)
Would prescribe NSAIDs	59.0	61.9	67.5	54.9	1.93 (1.39–2.66)
Advice on exercise	58.6	70.6	58.7	64.3	1.34 (0.96–1.86)
Advice on work modification	40.2	51.1	43.1	41.6	1.65 (1.20–2.27)
Specialist referral	2.9	0.7	2.0	3.7	0.13 (0.04–0.46)
Physiotherapy referral	52.2	51.8	53.4	56.5	0.87 (0.63–1.19)
Would not refer	38.5	41.8	42.2	34.4	1.60 (1.16–2.21)
Stated management of subacute low back pain					
Would not order tests	6.2	10.5	7.7	6.8	2.01 (1.11–3.65)
Would order lumbosacral X-rays	65.1	63.9	67.0	64.5	1.06 (0.76–1.48)
Special imaging (CT, MRI, myelogram)	37.8	30.3	35.9	39.1	0.62 (0.45–0.87)
Would prescribe bed rest	6.8	2.0	7.5	3.3	0.64 (0.27–1.52)
Would prescribe NSAIDs	66.3	71.5	71.3	66.4	1.61 (1.14–2.26)
Advice on exercise	47.3	57.5	50.3	53.1	1.34 (0.98–1.84)
Advice on work modification	44.0	56.6	52.7	50.0	1.85 (1.35–2.54)
Specialist referral	33.1	19.9	31.9	31.5	0.51 (0.36–0.73)
Physiotherapy referral	58.2	65.7	64.1	60.7	1.59 (1.15–2.20)
Would not refer	6.5	8.2	7.2	6.8	1.35 (0.74–2.49)

[1] Ratio of odds ratio – odds of change (either increased or decreased) in Victoria compared to NSW

1.65 times as likely to advise work modification. Similar changes were seen for subacute low back pain (Buchbinder *et al.*, 2001b).

Victorian WorkCover Authority claims database

Analysis of the Victorian WorkCover Authority claims database revealed that the number of back claims in comparison to non-back claims declined by greater than 15 per cent over the duration of the study (Buchbinder *et al.*, 2001a). This was accompanied by a decline in the rate of days compensated for back claims steeper than that seen for non-back claims and a 20 per cent reduction in medical payments per back claim seen over the duration of the campaign.

Follow-up population study

Repeat telephone surveys were recently performed in Victoria and New South Wales, 3 years after cessation of the campaign (Buchbinder and Jolley, 2004). To our knowledge, no public health interventions for back pain have taken place in either state since the end of 1999. A further 1500 surveys were completed: 900 in Victoria and 600 in NSW. Awareness of back pain advertising in Victoria declined between Surveys 3 and 4 (47.1, 73.9, 85.5, and 63.9 per cent at Surveys 1–4 respectively; p <0.0001) with no changes observed over time in NSW (51.2, 48.5, 48.0, and 50.8 per cent at Surveys 1–4 respectively).

Population beliefs about back pain in Victoria at Survey 4 were less positive when compared to survey 3, but were still significantly better than at baseline and higher than at Survey 2 (mean Back Beliefs Questionnaire scores 26.5, 28.4, 29.7, 28.8 at Surveys 1–4 respectively; Table 11.1). This was again observed irrespective of demographic factors. There was no change in New South Wales between successive surveys. As for the other time points, female gender, white collar occupation, higher education level, and income were all associated with better Back Beliefs Questionnaire scores (Table 11.5).

These data indicate that there has been a sustained positive shift in population beliefs about back pain in Victoria since cessation of the media campaign 3 years ago. This was again seen across the whole distribution of baseline back beliefs, indicating that these views may now be the accepted norm and less effort may be required to maintain this position and achieve long-term behavioural change (Rose, 1985; Buchbinder *et al.*, 2002). However there has been some decay in the observed effect between Surveys 3 and 4 and top-up reminders and/or other strategies may be necessary to maintain improvements over time. Follow-up general practitioner surveys are currently underway to determine whether there have also been sustained positive shifts in doctors' beliefs in Victoria.

Table 11.5 Influence of demographic factors on Back Beliefs Questionnaire (BBQ) Score in Victoria at Survey 4

Demographic factor	Category	N	Mean BBQ score
Age group	18–24	107	28.8
	25–34	225	28.6
	35–49	379	28.8
	50–65	189	28.9
Gender[1]	Male	450	28.2
	Female	450	29.4
Location	Melbourne	504	28.8
	Country Vic	396	28.7
Occupation[1]	Upper white-collar	83	31.0
	Lower white-collar	487	29.0
	Upper blue	172	28.4
	Lower blue	144	27.0
Highest level of education achieved[1]	Primary	213	27.0
	Secondary	237	28.6
	Diploma	143	28.9
	Degree	209	29.7
	Post-graduate	98	31.3
Australian-born[1]	Yes	722	29.1
	No	178	27.4
Employment status	Self-employed	125	28.7
	Manager	198	29.3
	Employee	571	28.6
Household Income[1]	<$20 K	41	26.8
	$20–30 K	87	27.5
	$30–40 K	115	28.5
	$40–50 K	106	27.9
	$50–60 K	120	28.6
	$60–70 K	65	28.5
	$70–80 K	51	29.6
	>$80 K	199	30.1
	Refused/didn't know	115	29.4

[1] Within group differences, $P < 0.05$

Managing disability by public policy initiatives

Based upon empirical data, we have demonstrated that a public policy initiative designed to influence population attitudes and beliefs about back pain can achieve a sustained change in patients' and health professionals' behaviour. The media campaign sought to promote positive beliefs about back pain, encourage self-coping strategies and continued activity, and reduce negative beliefs about the inevitable consequences of back pain. It provided the community with up-to-date and accurate information about back pain and its management and gave it the confidence to deal with back pain. It also empowered health professionals to manage back pain in a more appropriate fashion and persuaded employers to keep back pain sufferers at work.

There are compelling arguments for this approach (Buchbinder *et al.*, 2001c; Buchbinder *et al.*, 2002). As explained above, disability related to low back pain is a public health issue because it affects a substantial proportion of the community and involves the use of substantial common resources. Second, psychosocial interventions have been shown to reduce disability and work absence associated with low back trouble (Symonds *et al.*, 1995). These interventions aim to reduce the risk of chronicity by changing beliefs with concomitant behavioural modification leading to adoption of an early active management strategy (Burton *et al.*, 1996). The data suggest that informative interventions could even be of more value when initiated early, even prior to the onset of symptoms (Symonds *et al.*, 1995).

Third, predictive models of low back pain are not at present able to identify those at risk of disability. By targeting the entire population, a public health approach will reach those hard-to-identify, high-risk groups. There is also much evidence that a population strategy of universal change has greater overall effect than targeted high-risk strategies. Fourth, the population approach may be an effective way of modifying doctors' and other health professionals' behaviour, both through direct influences as well as through the change in attitudes of their patients. There is good evidence that doctors strive to please their patients, and that they are open to patients' requests to try treatments (Avorn *et al.*, 1982).

The 'direct-to-consumer' approach is recognized as a powerful force in pharmaceutical marketing, and it is likely that similarly effective results can be achieved by public health media campaigns as by drug company marketing schemes (Buchbinder *et al.*, 2002). With the current emphasis on consumerism in the delivery of health care, it is important to recognize that in the area of back pain, other competing interests in the area of back pain already use the mass media to convey their messages. This was illustrated in our studies by the fact that about 50 per cent of the general population and 15 to 25 per cent of general practitioners who responded to our surveys were aware of advertising campaigns about back pain prior to the onset of the Victorian WorkCover Authority media campaign in Victoria. Not only is it imperative that the reporting of health-related issues in the lay media correctly represent the best available knowledge on the effectiveness of health care interventions, it should also discourage use of interventions of unproven effectiveness. To succeed, mass media campaigns need to be up to date, clever, and attract the attention of the public. Finally, employer attitudes and beliefs and workplace philosophies may also be influenced through similar means.

Implications for health policy

It is hoped that the demonstration of effectiveness of the back pain media campaign will have important ramifications for further policy development in this area, as well as lead to innovative approaches to other health problems. Our results have encouraged others to implement similar back programmes. For example a major public education campaign, entitled 'Working Backs Scotland' was launched in Scotland in October 2000 (Health Education Board for Scotland (HEBS) and the Health and Safety Executive (HSE), 2000). Like the Victorian campaign, a key aim of this project is to encourage all professionals and therapists to deliver a consistent message to those who suffer from back pain and to help people with back pain understand how they can help themselves.

The success of the Australian social marketing campaign has also stimulated replication of the intervention in Alberta, Canada, through the support of the Workers Compensation Board – Alberta and others. It is believed the intervention will have the same dramatic effect on reducing disability and reliance on health care professionals for care of back pain in Alberta as it did in Australia. It will be important to determine whether the success of the Victorian campaign can be replicated in other industrialized societies with other health-care and disability systems and plans are underway to evaluate the success of the Alberta campaign.

Acknowledgements

Associate Professor Damien Jolley and Dr Mary Wyatt, co-investigators on the Victorian WorkCover Authority Evaluation Project.

References

Andersson G (1997). The epidemiology of spinal disorders. In: JW Frymoyer, ed. *The adult spine: principles and practice*, pp. 93–141. New York: Raven Press.

Avorn J, Chen M and Hartley R (1982). Scientific versus commercial sources of influence on the prescribing behavior of physicians. *American Journal of Medicine*, **73**, 4–8.

Battie MC, Cherkin DC, Dunn R, Ciol MA and Wheeler K (1994). Managing low back pain: attitudes and treatment preferences of physical therapists. *Physical Therapy*, **74**, 219–226.

Bero L, Grilli R, Grimshaw JM, Harvey E, Oxman AD and Thomson MA (1998). Closing the gap between research and practice: an overview of systematic reviews of interventions to promote the implementation of research findings. *British Medical Journal*, **317**, 465–468.

Bombardier C, Jansz G and Maetzel A (1995). Primary care physicians' knowledge, confidence and attitude in the management of acute low back pain. *Arthritis and Rheumatism*, **38** (suppl.), S385.

Bridges-Webb C, Britt H, Miles DA, Neary S, Charles J and Traynor V (1992). Morbidity and treatment in general practice in Australia 1990–1991. *Medical Journal of Australia*, **157** (suppl.), S1–S56.

Brooks P and Hart J (2000). The bone and joint decade: 2000–2010. *Medical Journal of Australia*, **172**, 307–308.

Buchbinder R and Jolley D (2004). Population-based intervention to change back pain beliefs: a three-year follow up study. *British Medical Journal*, **328**, 321.

Buchbinder R, Jolley D and Wyatt M (2001a). Population based intervention to change back pain beliefs and disability: three part evaluation. *British Medical Journal*, **322**, 1516–1520.

Buchbinder R, Jolley D and Wyatt M (2001b). Effects of a media campaign on back pain beliefs and its potential influence on management of low back pain in general practice. *Spine*, **26**, 2535–2542.

Buchbinder R, Jolley D and Wyatt M (2001c). Breaking the back of back pain. *Medical Journal of Australia*, **175**, 456–457.

Buchbinder R, Jolley D and Wyatt M (2002). Role of the media in disability management. In: T Sullivan and J Frank, eds. *Preventing and managing disabling injury at work*, pp. 101–141. Toronto: Taylor and Francis.

Burton AK, Tillotson KM, Main CJ and Hollis S (1995). Psychosocial predictors of outcome in acute and subchronic low back trouble. *Spine*, **20**, 722–728.

Burton A, Waddell G, Burtt R and Blair S (1996). Patient educational material in the management of low back pain in primary care. *Bulletin – Hospital for Joint Diseases*, **55**, 138–141.

Burton A, Waddell G, Tillotson KM and Summerton N (1999). Information and advice to patients with back pain can have a positive effect. A randomised controlled trial of a novel educational booklet in primary care. *Spine*, **24**, 1–8.

Carey T and Garrett J (1996). Patterns of ordering diagnostic tests for patients with acute low back pain. The North Carolina Back Pain Project. *Annals of Internal Medicine*, **125**, 807–814.

Carey TS, Garrett J, Jackman A, McLaughlin C, Fryer J and Smucker DR (1995). The outcomes and costs of care for acute low back pain among patients seen by primary care practitioners, chiropractors, and orthopedic surgeons. The North Carolina Back Pain Project. *New England Journal of Medicine*, **333**, 913–917.

Cherkin DC, Deyo RA, Street JH and Barlow W (1996). Predicting poor outcomes for back pain seen in primary care using patients' own criteria. *Spine*, **21**, 2900–2907.

Cherkin DC, Deyo RA, Wheeler K and Ciol MA (1995). Physician views about treating low back pain. The results of a national survey. *Spine*, **20**, 1–10.

Cherkin DC, MacCornack FA and Berg AO (1988). Managing low back pain – a comparison of the beliefs and behaviors of family physicians and chiropractors. *Western Journal of Medicine*, **149**, 475–480.

Chew-Graham C and May C (1997). The benefits of back pain. *Family Practice*, **14**, 461–465.

Chew-Graham C and May C (1999). Chronic low back pain in general practice: the challenge of the consultation. *Family Practice*, **16**, 46–49.

Croft PR, Macfarlane GJ, Papageorgiou AC, Thomas E and Silman AJ (1998). Outcome of low back pain in general practice: a prospective study. *British Medical Journal*, **316**, 1356–1359.

Cypress B (1983). Characteristics of physician visits for back pain symptoms: a national perspective. *American Journal of Public Health*, **73**, 389–395.

Deyo R (1996a). Drug therapy for back pain. Which drugs help which patients? *Spine*, **21**, 2840–2849.

Deyo R (1996b). Acute low back pain: a new paradigm for management. *British Medical Journal*, **313**, 1343–1344.

Deyo R and Diehl A (1986). Patient satisfaction with medical care for low-back pain. *Spine*, **11**, 28–30.

Deyo R, Diehl A and Rosenthal M (1987). Reducing roentgenography use. Can patient expectations be altered? *Archives of Internal Medicine*, **147**, 141–145.

Deyo R and Phillips W (1996). Low back pain. A primary care challenge. *Spine*, **21**, 2826–2832.

Dixon A (1990). The evolution of clinical policies. *Medical Care*, **28**, 201–220.

Elam K, Cherkin D and Deyo R (1995). How emergency physicians approach low back pain: choosing costly options. *Journal of Emergency Medicine*, **13**, 143–150.

Frank J, Sinclair S, Hogg-Johnson S, *et al.* (1998). Preventing disability from work-related low-back pain. New evidence gives new hope—if we can just get all the players onside. *Canadian Medical Association Journal*, **158**, 1625–1631.

Freeborn D, Shye D, Mullooly JP, Eraker S and Romeo J (1997). Primary care physicians' use of lumbar spine imaging tests. Effects of guidelines and practice pattern feedback. *Journal of General Internal Medicine*, **12**, 619–625.

Grilli R, Ramsey C and Minozzi S (2002). Mass media interventions: effects on health services utilisation. *Cochrane Database of Systematic Reviews*, **1**, CD000389.

Hart L, Deyo RA and Cherkin DC (1995). Physician office visits for low back pain. Frequency, clinical evaluation, and treatment patterns from a U.S. national survey. *Spine*, **20**, 11–19.

Health Education Board for Scotland (HEBS) and the Health and Safety Executive (HSE) (2000). *Working backs Scotland*. Available at: http://www.workingbacksscotland.com/.

Hendler N (1984). Depression caused by chronic pain. *Journal of Clinical Psychiatry*, **45**, 30–36.

Hill D, White V, Marks R and Boland R (1993). Changes in sun-related attitudes and behaviours, and reduced sunburn prevalence in a population at high risk of melanoma. *European Journal of Cancer Prevention*, **2**, 447–456.

Indahl A, Velund L and Reikeraas O (1995). Good prognosis for low back pain when left untampered. A randomized clinical trial. *Spine*, **20**, 473–477.

Industry Commission Report (1995). *Work safety and health: an inquiry into occupational health and safety*. Commonwealth of Australia.

Klenerman L, Slade PD, Stanley M, *et al.* (1995). The prediction of chronicity in patients with an acute attack of low back pain in a general practice setting. *Spine*, **20**, 478–484.

Kravitz R, Callahan EJ, Paterniti D, Antonius D, Dunham M and Lewis CE (1997). Prevalence and sources of patients' unmet expectations for care. *Annals of Internal Medicine*, **125**, 730–737.

Lethem J, Slade PD, Troup JD and Bentley G (1983). Outline of a fear avoidance model of exaggerated pain perception. Part 1. *Behaviour Research and Therapy*, **21**, 401–408.

Linton SJ (2000). A review of psychological risk factors in back and neck pain. *Spine*, **25**, 1148–1156.

Little P, Cantrell T, Roberts L, Chapman J, Langridge J and Pickering R (1998). Why do GPs perform investigations?: the medical and social agendas in arranging back X-rays. *Family Practice*, **15**, 264–265.

Little P, Smith L, Cantrell T, Chapman J, Langridge J and Pickering R (1996). General practitioners' management of acute back pain: a survey of reported practice compared with clinical guidelines. *British Medical Journal*, **312**, 485–488.

Loeser J and Sullivan M (1995). Disability in the chronic low back pain patient may be iatrogenic. *Pain Forum*, **4**, 114–121.

Loisel P, Abenhaim, L, Durand P, *et al.* (1997). A population-based, randomized clinical trial on back pain management. *Spine*, **22**, 2911–2918.

Maetzel A, Johnson SH, Woodbury M and Bombardier C (2000). Use of grade membership analysis to profile the practice styles of individual physicians in the management of acute low back pain. *Journal of Clinical Epidemiology*, **53**, 195–205.

Malmivaara A, Häkkinen U, Aro T, *et al.* (1995). The treatment of acute low back pain – bed rest, exercises, or ordinary activity? *New England Journal of Medicine*, **332**, 351–355.

Marks R (1999). Two decades of the public health approach to skin cancer control in Australia: Why, how, and where are we now? *Australasian Journal of Dermatology*, **40**, 1–5.

Mathers C and Penn R (1999). *Health system costs of injury, poisoning and musculo-skeletal disorders in Australia 1993–94*. Canberra: Australian Institute of Health and Welfare.

Nachemson A, Waddell G and Norlund AI (2000). Epidemiology of neck and back pain. In: A Nachemson and E Jonsson, eds. *Neck and back pain. The scientific evidence of causes, diagnosis, and treatment*, pp. 165–188. Philadelphia: Lippincott Williams and Wilkins.

Ostelo RW, Stomp-van den Berg SG, Vlaeyen J W, Wolters PM and de Vet HC (2003). Health care provider's attitudes and beliefs towards chronic low back pain: the development of a questionnaire. *Manual Therapy*, **8**, 214–222.

Owen JP, Rutt G, Keir MJ, Spencer H, Richardson D, Richardson A and Barclay C (1990). Survey of general practitioners' opinions on the role of radiology in patients with low back pain. *British Journal of General Practice*, **40**, 98–101.

Owen N, Bauman A, Booth M, Oldenburg M and Magnus P (1995). Serial mass-media campaigns to promote physical activity: reinforcing or redundant? *American Journal of Public Health*, **85**, 244–248.

Philips H and Jahanshahi M (1986). The components of pain behaviour report. *Behaviour Research and Therapy*, **24**, 117–125.

Phillips D, Kanter ES, Bednarczyk B and Tastad PL (1991). Importance of the lay press in the transmission of medical knowledge to the scientific community. *New England Journal of Medicine*, **325**, 1180–1183.

Pierce J, Macaskill P and Hill D (1990). Long-term effectiveness of mass media led anti-smoking campaigns in Australia. *American Journal of Public Health*, **80**, 565–569.

Rainville J, Carlson N, Polatin, P, Gatchel RJ and Indahl A (2000). Exploration of physicians' recommendations for activities in chronic low back pain. *Spine*, **25**, 2210–2220.

Redman S, Spencer E and Sanson-Fisher R (1990). The role of mass media in changing health-related behaviour: a critical appraisal of two methods. *Health Promotion International*, **5**, 85–101.

Roland M and Dixon M (1989). Randomised controlled trial of an educational booklet for patients presenting with back pain in general practice. *Journal of the Royal College of General Practitioners*, **39**, 244–246.

Roland M, Waddell G, Moffat JK, Burton K, Main C and Cantrell T (1996). *The back book*. UK: The Stationary Office.

Rose G (1985). Sick individuals and sick populations. *International Journal of Epidemiology*, **30**, 427–432.

Rossignol M, Abenhaim L, Séguin P, Neveu A, Collet JP, Ducruet T and Shapiro S (2000). Coordination of primary health care for back pain. A randomized controlled trial. *Spine*, **25**, 251–259.

Schiottz-Christensen B, Nielsen GL, Hansen VK, Schodt T, Sorensen HT and Olesen F (1999). Long-term prognosis of acute low back pain in patients seen in general practice: a 1-year prospective follow-up study. *Family Practice*, **16**, 223–232.

Schroth W, Schectman JM, Elinsky EG and Panagides JC (1992). Utilization of medical services for the treatment of acute low back pain: conformance with clinical guidelines. *Journal of General Internal Medicine*, **7**, 486–491.

Skelton A, Murphy EA, Murphy RS and O'Dowd TC (1996). Patients' views of low back pain and its management in general practice. *British Journal of General Practice*, **46**, 153–156.

Sly D, Hopkins RS, Trapido E and Ray S (2001). Influence of a counteradvertising media campaign on initiation of smoking: The Florida 'truth' Campaign. *American Journal of Public Health*, **91**, 233–238.

Symonds TL, Burton AK, Tillotson KM and Main CJ (1995). Absence resulting from low back trouble can be reduced by psychosocial intervention at the work place. *Spine*, **20**, 2738–2744.

Symonds TL, Burton AK, Tillotson KM and Main CJ (1996). Do attitudes and beliefs influence work loss due to low back trouble? *Occupational Medicine*, **46**, 25–32.

van den Hoogen HJ, Koes BW, van Eijk JT, Bouter LM and Deville W (1998). On the course of low back pain in general practice: a one year follow up study. *Annals of the Rheumatic Diseases*, **57**, 13–19.

van der Weide WE, Verbeek JH and van Tulder MW (1997). Vocational outcome of intervention for low-back pain. *Scandinavian Journal of Work, Environment and Health*, **23**, 165–178.

van Tulder M, Croft P, van Splunteren P, *et al.* (2002). Disseminating and implementing the results of back pain research in primary care. *Spine*, **27**, E121–127.

van Tulder M, Koes B and Bouter L (1997). Conservative treatment of acute and chronic nonspecific low back pain. A systematic review of randomized controlled trials of the most common interventions. *Spine*, **22**, 2128–2156.

Victorian WorkCover Authority (2001). In: *Annual Report Victorian WorkCover Authority 1999/2000*. Melbourne, Vic.

Victorian WorkCover Authority (1996). *Guidelines for the management of employees with compensable low back pain*. Melbourne: Victorian WorkCover Authority.

von Korff M (1994). Studying the natural history of back pain. *Spine*, **19**, 2041–2045.

von Korff M, Barlow W, Cherkin D and Deyo R (1994). Effects of practice style in managing back pain. *Annals of Internal Medicine*, **121**, 187–195.

Waddell G (1987). 1987 Volvo award in clinical sciences. A new clinical model for the treatment of low-back pain. *Spine*, **12**, 632–644.

Waddell G, Feder G and Lewis M (1997). Systematic reviews of bed rest and advice to stay active for acute low back pain. *British Journal of General Practice*, **47**, 647–652.

Waddell G, Newton M, Henderson I, Somerville D and Main CJ (1993). A fear-avoidance beliefs questionnaire (FABQ) and the role of fear-avoidance beliefs in chronic low back pain and disability. *Pain*, **52**, 157–168.

Wensig M, van der Weijden T and Grol R (1998). Implementing guidelines and innovations in general practice: which interventions are effective? *British Journal of General Practice*, **48**, 991–997.

Zarkowska E and Philips H (1986). Recent onset vs. persistent pain: evidence for a distinction. *Pain*, **25**, 365–372.

Chapter 12

Clinician bias in diagnosis and treatment

Duncan B. Double

Introduction

The history of medicine has been said to be largely the history of the placebo effect (Houston, 1938). Doctors' beliefs and hopes about treatment, combined with patients' suggestibility, may have an apparent therapeutic effect. Countless ailments throughout history have seemingly been relieved by medicines and other medical interventions because sufferers and their doctors have believed in them.

There can be disastrous consequences from patients investing their faith in the omnipotence of doctors. As an example, I want to look at the notorious case of the Kaadt diabetic clinic, founded on the 'wonderful new treatment' for diabetes initially marketed by Dr Charles Kaadt. This promise of a new cure was made available soon after Frederick G. Banting was awarded the Nobel prize, in 1923, for the discovery of insulin. Kaadt's formula was essentially saltpetre – potassium nitrate – dissolved in vinegar. Nonetheless, he told his patients that an old European woman disclosed the secret of the formula to him.

James Harvey Young (1992) tells the story of the two Kaadt brothers, Charles and Peter, in a chapter of his book *The Medical Messiahs*. Both doctors made considerable sums of money because of their diabetic treatment, but lost their licences to practice. Young's book demonstrates that quackery in America persisted despite the passing of the first Food and Drugs Act in 1906. He gives some indication of why quack remedies for diabetes may have had such appeal.

> [D]iabetes, before insulin, could be treated only with a regimen of hygiene and severely circumscribed diet, both as to quantity and kinds of food. Although semi-starving lengthened the life expectancy, patients often rebelled against its limitations and yielded to the quack's promise of an easier way.

> (Young, 1992, p. 218)

Even after insulin therapy was introduced, as Young notes,

> [t]he only method of introducing insulin into the body was by hypodermic injection –
> in the early years by several injections a day. Quacks, in playing on fear of the needle,
> struck a responsive chord.
>
> (Young, 1992, p. 219)

There were many satisfied users of the Kaadt therapy. Even at the 1948 trial of the Kaadt brothers and their clinic superintendent, defence witnesses told of remarkable recoveries. Despite this evidence, the Kaadt brothers were convicted of violating the 1938 Food and Drugs law by giving false and misleading information about the efficacy of their treatment.

The Kaadt brothers did not subscribe to the orthodox explanation of diabetes as pancreatic insufficiency of insulin. Instead, they believed that their treatment corrected a digestive problem. The standard treatment for insulin was therefore wrong and they advised patients to give up their insulin treatment. This abandonment of proper treatment was clearly the most dangerous feature of their advice.

The Kaadt brothers were obviously not merely misunderstood scientists, as their defence attorney suggested in his summing up of the trial. Such is the self-protective power of denial that it is likely at the trial that Peter Kaadt still believed that diabetes was due to poor digestion. He left the witness stand after cross-examination 'apparently near breakdown'. Charles Kaadt sat through the trial showing little interest in what went on. He said he had been very sick and could remember hardly anything. The judge may well have been correct that the Kaadt brothers had engaged 'in a sordid, an evil and a vicious enterprise, without the slightest regard or consideration for the patients that consulted [them]'.

What I want to highlight from this case is the powerful combination of gullible patients and misinformed doctors. The Kaadt brothers could only have succeeded if they had enough believers in their treatment, but their theory about diabetes was totally wrong. How much of the theories of modern medicine are incorrect? What biases do doctors still introduce into the processes of diagnosis and treatment?

Illness is one of the key problems of life. It may not be surprising that we take an antirational approach to dealing with it. We want a simple, quick, cheap, painless, and complete cure. If the science of medicine could ever win a total victory over disease, then we would not have any need for pseudoscience. To quote from Skrabanek and McCormick's (1998) *Follies and fallacies in medicine*:

> The physician's belief in his treatment and the patient's faith in his physician exert a
> mutually reinforcing effect; the result is a powerful remedy which is almost guaranteed
> to produce an improvement and sometimes a cure. As a rule, discussions of the

placebo effect concentrate on the gullibility of patients but ignore the self-deception of physicians. . . . Patients who receive treatment are readily persuaded that they are having appropriate therapy and doctors may be deluded into believing that their prescribing is having specific effects. This results in a 'folie a deux' afflicting patient and doctor alike.

In this chapter, I want to attempt to correct the imbalance referred to by Skrabanek and McCormick by concentrating on misinformed doctors. The tendency for doctors to overvalue the verity of their clinical diagnosis and treatment is a major factor contributing to the placebo effect. Are doctors facing up to the extent to which their treatments may be placebos?

I want look briefly at medical error, and particular the diagnostic bias created through not taking psychosocial factors sufficiently into account. I move on to look at the implications for treatment, particularly overmedication of symptoms. The basis of decision-making about prescribing is discussed, with particular reference to the role of doctors' expectations. Finally, I want to look at the power of suggestion and to question whether expectancy has really been eliminated in the assessment of the efficacy of medical treatment.

Medical error and bias to make a physical diagnosis

Mistakes occur in medicine as much as in any other field. We are all fallible, and it is impossible for anybody to avoid all mistakes, even avoidable ones. This state of affairs was recognized by Neil McIntyre and Sir Karl Popper (1983) when they called for a new ethics in medicine. They proposed that doctors should avoid hypocrisy by not hiding mistakes. Nonetheless, the clinical task should still be to minimize errors in practice.

There have been several major inquiries in the NHS over recent years in the context of what appear to be medical errors and service failures (Walshe and Higgins, 2002). Inquires have become an increasingly common managerial and political response to a clinical governance incident. For example, since 1994, health authorities have been obliged to hold an independent inquiry in cases of homicides committed by those who have been in contact with the psychiatric services (Buchanan, 1999). The findings of inquiries seem to highlight similar sorts of institutional failures, which may suggest there are inherent difficulties in the system of medical practice.

I want to mention one inquiry for the purpose of my theme of misinformed doctors. This is the case of Dr Andrew Holton, previously consultant paediatrician at Leicester Royal Infirmary (Chadwick and Smith, 2002). He was suspended and referred to the General Medical Council. A review concluded that he had over-diagnosed and over-treated epilepsy in children (Royal College of Paediatrics and Child Health, 2001). Although regarded as a hard working and conscientious doctor, with a particular interest in Landau–Klefner syndrome, the report by the British Paediatric Neurological Association found that Dr Holton went beyond the available evidence in his belief that epilepsy could account for many neurodevelopmental problems in children and that early aggressive treatment achieved better long-term outcome.

This verdict has to be set in the clinical context of the generally not uncommon over-diagnosis and over-treatment of epilepsy in clinical practice. Holton's practice could be seen as being at the extreme of a continuum. For example 39 per cent of children admitted as inpatients in 1997 to the Danish Epilepsy Centre for Children did not have epilepsy (Uldall *et al.*, 2001). Similarly, 38 per cent of children re-evaluated at a tertiary centre in Sarajevo were found not to have epilepsy (Zubcevic *et al.*, 2001). Diagnosis of epilepsy can be challenging. Differential diagnosis includes pseudoseizures, ranging from syncope to psychogenic events. Over-diagnosis may therefore be frequent.

In the case of Dr Andrew Holton, although he may have had certain idiosyncrasies in his diagnostic style, a considerable proportion of the blame was placed on system errors such as insufficient training, being overworked, and being isolated from specialist support. The general tendency in clinical governance has been to concentrate on system errors in complex health care systems (Cook *et al.*, 2000).

I want to suggest that Dr Andrew Holton is the, not unexpected, outcome of a medical system that overestimates the potential for physical intervention. This is a system error that investigations into the case of Andrew Horton have not sufficiently considered. In fact, the independent review of paediatric neurology services in Leicester, where Dr Holton worked, established by the Regional Director of Public Health, did not even attempt to judge Dr Holton's clinical practice (Department of Health, 2003). This aspect is left to the medical profession, but professional attitudes may not be sufficiently unbiased. Doctors may find it difficult to acknowledge the extent to which they themselves are therapeutic agents for the placebo effect.

I am focusing on bias, which is a term that refers to systematic deviation from validity, or to some deformation of practice that produces such deviation. Bias tends to produce spurious results whereas random error may obscure true conclusions. Medicine needs to be more aware of its own self-deception.

In particular, I want to look at the bias produced by clinician **over**-diagnosis and **over**-treatment, in the way that Dr Horton over-diagnosed and over-treated epilepsy. Of course, in the ordinary course of their practice doctors both under- and over-diagnose. However, I think it is difficult to find evidence of a bias for under-diagnosis, in the sense of a systematic error as I have just defined it. Under-diagnosis seems to be idiosyncratic and dependent on individual clinicians. This random error also affects over-diagnosis, but I think in addition there is evidence of a systematic bias for over-diagnosis. And I will argue that this bias is related to the conceptual framework of a biomedical way of looking at practice.

False-positive diagnoses for other disorders besides epilepsy are also quite common. Let me give three examples:

1 The diagnosis of heart failure was unconfirmed by echocardiography in 48 per cent of patients receiving diuretics for presumptive heart failure, particularly in women (Wheeldon *et al.*, 1993).

2 The diagnosis of cerebrovascular disease was unmade in 27 per cent of cases of transient ischaemic attack (TIA) and minor stroke referred to a regional neurovascular centre (Martin *et al.*, 1997).

3 Providing treatment for pulmonary embolism (PE) without objective confirmation of an embolus was regarded as preferable to missing a case of PE in a utility analysis of physicians' attitude towards misdiagnosis of PE before ordering lung scanning (Rosen *et al.*, 2000).

Patients may well not be aware that the level of over-diagnosis of such common conditions as heart failure and cerebrovascular disease is so high. I want to suggest that there is a common theme in the examples I have given. For example it may be easier to diagnose heart failure and cerebrovascular disease than to attempt to disentangle the emotional origins of non-specific symptoms that may mimic cardiac and cerebrovascular disease. Misdiagnosing pseudoepilepsy as epilepsy suggests that the problem arises because of concentration on a disease model of diagnosis. Pseudoepilepsy may not have a physical pathological basis. Yet doctors tend to be looking for the physical cause of patients' symptoms.

Doctors tend to err on the side of caution, as witnessed by the pulmonary embolism example. It is more of a 'crime' to miss a physical diagnosis than to create a non-disease. But overall diagnosis needs to take psychosocial factors into account. Failure to do so may lead to an over-diagnosis of physical disease, and may miss psychosocial diagnoses. Over-diagnosis may therefore arise through taking an overly physical perspective of the presentation of symptoms. Medicine's search for physical causes leads to a surfeit of positive diagnoses.

To examine this issue further, I want to look more generally at so-called medically unexplained symptoms. 'Medically unexplained symptoms' is a term that has gained recent popularity. Its meaning is little different from other similar terms used previously, such as functional, hysterical, and somatoform disorders. These labels are applied to symptoms for which doctors cannot find a physical cause. By examining how readily doctors are prepared to apply the term medically unexplained symptoms, we may detect a bias in favour of making a physical diagnosis.

Medically explained symptoms and psychosocial factors in diagnosis

Doctors, perhaps particularly in general practice, are confronted with a diversity of symptoms that do not necessarily conform with neat textbook descriptions of diagnoses. GPs operate in an atmosphere of low disease prevalence and deal with a high incidence of non-specific symptoms. It has been estimated that about 70 to 90 per cent of general practice patients are without serious physical disorder (Barsky, 1981). Medically unexplained symptoms are also common in secondary care. About 50 per cent of patients meet such criteria across a range of outpatient clinics, with medically unexplained symptoms being the most common diagnosis in some specialities (Nimnuan *et al.*, 2001).

Nimnuan *et al.* (2000) studied the accuracy of doctors' provisional diagnosis of medically unexplained illness. Physicians were asked to state whether they thought the patients' presenting symptoms were medically explained or medically unexplained. Subsequent case notes were examined to determine whether investigations or later examinations revealed an explained cause of patients' symptoms. Congruence between the final diagnosis and the physicians' provisional diagnosis are shown in Table 12.1.

These results show that doctors are more likely to change their provisional diagnosis from medically explained to medically unexplained (56 per cent) rather than the reverse of changing from medically unexplained to explained (17 per cent). In other words, on initial presentation they over-diagnose what turn out to be medically unexplained symptoms as a physical diagnosis. This suggests they worry more about errors of omission rather than commission,

Table 12.1 Congruence between physicians' provisional and final diagnosis

Provisional diagnosis	Final diagnosis	
	Medically unexplained	**Medically explained**
Medically unexplained	118 (44%)	43 (17%)
Medically explained	152 (56%)	213 (83%)
Total	270 (100%)	256 (100%)

leading to potential over-diagnosis of physical disease and over-investigation of psychosocial symptoms.

This demonstration of the under-diagnosis of medically unexplained symptoms is reminiscent of the reported under-recognition of psychiatric disorders in general practice, and medical practice in general. Research suggests that general practitioners fail to diagnose up to half of cases of depression or anxiety on initial presentation (Goldberg and Huxley, 1992). Over the longer term this figure may not be as high or as clinically important as this initial impression may suggest (Kessler *et al.*, 2002). Some depressed patients are given a diagnosis at subsequent consultations or recover without a general practitioner's diagnosis. However, there is still a significant minority of patients (14 per cent in this study) with a diagnosis of persistent depression that are undetected.

The failure of detection of depression is commonly presumed to arise because of a lack of psychological mindedness amongst doctors. What I am suggesting is that there is a bias towards making a physical diagnosis rather than a psychosocial diagnosis in medicine. This is understandable, considering the origin of modern medicine in the anatomo-clinical method and clinico-pathological correlation. It also makes sense for doctors to be cautious as patients consult them because they do not want a physical diagnosis to be missed. However, in general, objective evidence of disease is valued over subjective experience. Such a tendency creates a bias towards the over-diagnosis of physical illness.

Critical psychiatry

This bias extends beyond physical medicine to psychiatry. Although psychiatry deals with mental disorders, the origins of these disorders are not necessarily conceptualized in psychosocial terms. In particular, the biomedical model of mental illness postulates that abnormalities of brain functioning are the cause of mental illness (Roth and Kroll, 1986). There may have been a time when psychological approaches, such as psychoanalysis or the pragmatic psychobiology of Adolf Meyer (Winters, 1951/2), were more influential, but the biomedical approach currently dominates psychiatric practice.

Neurobiological approaches emphasize brain and genetic abnormalities as the basis for mental illness. The complexity of psychosocial meaning may, therefore, be oversimplified in psychiatric diagnosis and physical treatment. Application of the biomedical model creates controversy because of the potential to lead to objectification of the mentally ill (Double, 2002). At its most extreme, the biomedical approach reduces people to objects that need their biology cured.

A bias towards concentrating on biological causes may be particularly obvious in psychiatry, because the mental health field evidently relates to psychosocial aspects. What I am suggesting is that this bias is the same in the rest of medicine. Clearly there are biological correlates of disease in medicine and psychiatry, but psychosocial factors are also important. These may be dominant in some presentations, perhaps particularly psychiatric presentations. There needs to be more of a balanced perspective, or medical interventions may be inappropriately applied in situations where the real issues are psychosocial.

Over-treatment and polypharmacy

Having considered over-diagnosis, I want to move on to examine over-treatment. Bias that affects medical diagnosis is likely to have consequences for treatment.

Prescribing costs have been increasing rapidly over recent years. For example, in the UK, the increase in primary care drugs spending from 1998/99 to 2001/2 was 29 per cent compared to an increase of 21 per cent in total Family Health Services expenditure in the same period (Audit Commission, 2003). British GPs are usually described as conservative in their prescribing (Gilley, 1994). In the US, prescription drug expenditure has risen 15 per cent or more per year over the past several years (National Institute for Health Care Management, 2002). While spending on prescription drugs accounts for around 10 per cent of spending on health in the US, drug costs have in recent years contributed disproportionately to a sharp upturn in overall health costs.

Despite being in the era of evidence-based medicine, there has been a steady increase in the therapeutic options for a widening variety of indications, some with only marginal benefit (Pillans and Roberts, 1999). Thirty-five years ago there were approximately 600 medications readily available to patients, but it is now estimated that there are up to 8000 different pills, potions, and powders on the market (Berenbeim, 2002).

A report by the Audit Commission in 1994 suggested that irrational and inconsistent prescribing by British general practitioners costs the NHS over £400 m a year (Audit Commission, 1994). Particular evidence for polypharmacy, or the use of several drugs when fewer may be sufficient, comes from medication use in the elderly. This over-prescribing still seems to be increasing. For example cross-sectional surveys in Finland of people over 64 found that the number of people with concomitant use of over five medications (defined as polypharmacy) had increased between 1990–1 and 1998–9 from 19 to 25 per cent (Linjakumpu et al, 2002).

Three examples of over-prescribing and polypharmacy are given below:

1 Many patients with apparent treated, uncomplicated, mild to moderate hypertension do not need antihypertensive treatment and can be withdrawn from their therapy without developing persistent hypertension (Myers *et al*, 1996). This may be because some patients have been inappropriately started on medication merely because of transient increases in blood pressure measured at the doctor's office.

2 Antiepileptics are overused in the following situations: combination therapy when optimal treatment is with a single drug; long-term use (or continuation) in situations where it is not indicated (e.g. in children with simple febrile seizures); unnecessarily fast dose escalation rates; and unnecessarily high maintenance dosages (Perucca, 2002).

3 Up to 25 per cent of outpatients with schizophrenia may be receiving antipsychotic polypharmacy, usually consisting of both an atypical and a conventional agent. This is partly because a significant number of patients become 'stuck' on the combination when an attempt is made to switch medication to the newer atypical agent (Tapp *et al*, 2003).

Many other examples could be given. What I have tried to demonstrate is that there is a bias for over-diagnosis and over-treatment of patients' physical symptoms. This may arise out of an emphasis on bodily processes rather than fully integrating psychosocial factors, including medically unexplained symptoms. I want to move on to examine in more detail the reasons for over-prescribing by a micro-analysis of the decision by the doctor to prescribe. What pressures and influences have a bearing on the process of prescribing?

Patients' expectations and doctors' perception of patients' expectations

Over-prescribing is commonly blamed on the expectations of patients. My emphasis is on the role that the doctor plays in this exchange and the biases that the doctor's faith and belief in the treatment produces. This is an interesting, complicated interaction. Clearly, doctors cannot entirely blame patients for their over-prescribing (Britten, 1995). For example a significant number of prescriptions are not consumed, or even dispensed, suggesting that prescribing levels actually exceed patients' expectations. And, non-compliance with doctors' orders is commonly seen as a problem in its own right by doctors. Patients would not define it as a problem if their wish for medication were taken as the over-riding factor.

Studies of patient preferences have found that about a quarter of patients come to a consultation in primary care wanting a prescription (Little *et al*, 2001). Most patients (54 per cent) are 'neutral' about wanting a prescription. The term 'want' is quite a strong indication of preference. Measurement of patient expectation is affected by the question asked and the methodology used. Other studies have found higher figures of patients expecting or hoping for a prescription (50–67 per cent) using questions with a forced yes/no answer. Nonetheless, not all consultations seem to be motivated by the aim of acquiring a prescription from the doctor.

Although patients' expectation does correlate with actual prescribing, the doctors' perception of patients' expectations is the stronger determinant of the decision to prescribe (Cockburn and Pit, 1997; Britten and Ukoumunne, 1997). For the most part, doctors' and patients' expectations are in accord, although not always so. Patients still receive a prescription when they do not hope for one and conversely do not receive when they come to the consultation hoping for one.

Furthermore, Britten and Ukoumunne (1997) found that doctors considered 22 per cent of prescriptions that they wrote were not strictly indicated. Only 66 per cent of prescriptions were both clinically indicated from the doctors' perspective and hoped for by patients. This suggests there is scope for reducing prescribing without depriving patients of drugs they either need or want, although only 3 per cent of prescriptions were neither indicated nor hoped for.

The writing of non-indicated prescriptions was primarily associated with the doctors' sense of feeling pressurized. Bradley (1992) has studied the related issue of 'uncomfortable prescribing'. Antibiotics, tranquillizers or hypnotics, and symptomatic remedies are the drugs whose prescription most often lead to feelings of discomfort. The main reasons for feeling uncomfortable are concern about drug toxicity, failure to live up to the GPs' own expectations and concern about the inappropriateness of treatment, and ignorance or uncertainty. Respiratory tract infections were found to be by far the commonest conditions in incidents when the doctor feels uncomfortable. This is because most such infections are viral and not bacteriological in origin, and therefore will not respond to antibiotics.

In summary, I have concentrated on the actual process of the decision to prescribe in an attempt to elucidate the factors involved in the bias to overprescribe. The interaction between patients' and doctors' expectations may be complicated, but there is clear evidence that doctors themselves do have a role in producing a distortion of prescribing.

The importance of suggestion

Having looked at the psychological factors involved in the decision to prescribe, I want to return to the more general theme of this chapter, and the book overall, about the degree to which non-specific belief factors play a role in medicine. Despite the growth of scientific medicine, and the modern emphasis on evidence-based medicine, have we really eliminated useless, and possibly dangerous, medicines from clinical practice?

Progress was made with the introduction of clinical trial methodology, initially by the use of placebo controls and the single-blind method, and finally in the 1950s by the acceptance of the double-blind method (Bull, 1959). The extent to which doctors did not want to give up their placebogenic function is demonstrated by the considerable resistance to the introduction of the randomized, controlled trial. Many regarded it as an intrusion on medical practice (e.g. Nash, 1962). Eventually rigorous clinical trials were required by the authorities before approving applications for new drugs. However, the regulatory agencies themselves do not always maintain independence and are heavily reliant on the pharmaceutical industry (Abraham, 2002). Drug development and regulation is not merely a matter of technical science. Too often the balance of scientific doubt are weighed in the interests of manufacturers rather than patients and public health.

There is clear evidence that publication bias by the drug companies has biased the perception of effectiveness in the literature. For example Kirsch *et al.* (2002) used the Freedom of Information Act to obtain the New Drug Application (NDA) data sets from the US Food and Drug Administration for the six most widely prescribed antidepressants approved between 1987 and 1999. Analysing these studies produced a lower effect size for antidepressants than has generally been found. More than half of these clinical trials sponsored by the pharmaceutical companies failed to find significant drug/placebo differences. A similar finding of selective publication by drug companies for antidepressants was also found in data submitted to the Swedish regulatory authority (Melander *et al.*, 2003).

The limitations of double-blind trials are not always fully appreciated. In particular, they are not as double-blind as is commonly assumed. Assessors' guesses made after the end of treatment to determine whether subjects had been in the active or placebo arm of the trial are generally greater than chance (Shapiro and Shapiro, 1997). This implies that trials are not truly masked. Patients and doctors may be cued in to whether patients are taking active or placebo medication by a variety of means. In fact if treatment is clearly superior to placebo, this should be obvious to raters in the trial, making it not technically blind. Patients in clinical trials are naturally curious to ascertain whether they are in the active or placebo group, and may, for example, notice that placebo tablets they have been taking taste differently from medication to which they have previously become accustomed. Active medication may produce side-effects which distinguishes it from inert medication.

For example publications have reported that the ability of raters and subjects to distinguish placebo and antidepressant is greater than chance (Even et al, 2000). Degree of unmasking can be correlated with apparent antidepressant effect. Antidepressant trials, because they involve assessment of depression on rating scales, are particularly prone to the effects of unblinding, compared to trials which have endpoints, such as mortality, which are not so dependent on subjective assessment by raters.

The breaking of the double-blind on occasions has been interpreted as the explanation for a positive trial result. For example Karlowski et al. (1975) found that ascorbic acid seemed to reduce the duration of a common cold, but these differences were eliminated when taking into account the correct guesses of medication. If such an analysis can be produced to support sceptical views about the effectiveness of ascorbic acid, why should it not be applied to agents which are believed to have therapeutic potency, such as antidepressants?

In fact, mean-end-point differences found in clinical trials are often quite small on average. Continuing the example of using the data on antidepressants, from the FDA data analysed by Kirsch et al. (2002) it was found that the average difference between antidepressants and placebo in these trials was two points on the Hamilton Rating Scale for Depression. The Hamilton Scale is the most commonly used measure of depression, with a total score of 50 or 62, depending on which version is used. A difference of two points seems of doubtful clinical relevance.

These small differences reinforce the view that statistically positive results in some trials may merely be the consequence of an amplified placebo effect made apparent because of unmasking. The problem is that the results of 'double-blind' studies tend to be automatically accepted as scientifically valid. A misleading self-deception is encouraged that trials can be conducted completely double-blind and the role of expectancies is thereby underestimated.

Conclusion

In this chapter, essentially, I have been asking how much modern medicine is still infused by 'quackery'. I know there will be objections. After all, quacks were transparent impostors and charlatans and knew their cures were fraudulent. There is no such obvious deceit in modern medicine.

However, the sharp division between mainstream medicine and quackery is misleading (Porter, 2000). Regular practitioners have cashed in on commercial practices barely distinguishable from what has been regarded as quackery. The example of the Kaadt brothers, that started the chapter, shows that to some extent quacks may have believed in their remedies. Do the modern pharmaceutical companies really believe in their marketable drugs, or even care whether they are effective? If they did, would they not be concerned to eliminate the bias that is still present in clinical trials? It is widely accepted that clinical trials cannot be conducted double-blind, but the pretence continues that the effectiveness of modern medicines has been proven.

I have suggested that medicine's concern with physical causes produces a relative neglect of personal and psychosocial aspects of illness. This attitude reinforces medicine's tendency to deny its placebo effect and, in practice, leads to a bias for over-diagnosis and over-treatment of physical conditions.

Despite my critique, there may be some reason for optimism. Over recent years, there have been attempts to transform the clinical method and develop the patient-centred model of care (Stewart *et al.*, 2003). The aim is to replace the traditional disease-centred method of care. Of course, being patient-centred does not mean doctors giving up being experts in the pathophysiology of disease. But patients also expect doctors to be experts in the experience of illness.

In a way, what I am saying is that clinician bias in diagnosis and treatment may be counteracted by patient-centred medicine. The influence of the doctor–patient relationship needs to become more open, so that doctors are not deceiving their patients. This has to start with them becoming more aware of their own bias. The aim of this chapter has been to try and improve that awareness.

References

Abraham J (2002). The pharmaceutical industry as a political player. *Lancet*, **360**, 1498–1502.

Audit Commission (1994). *A prescription for improvement – towards more rational prescribing in general practice*. London: Audit Commission/HMSO.

Audit Commission (2003). *Primary care prescribing. A bulletin for primary care trusts*. London: Audit Commission.

Barsky AJ (1981). Hidden reasons why some patients visit doctors. *Annals of Internal Medicine*, **94**, 492–498.

Berenbeim DM (2002). Polypharmacy: Overdosing on good intentions. *Managed Care Quarterly*, **10**, 1–5.

Bradley CP (1992). Uncomfortable prescribing decisions: A critical incident study. *British Medical Journal*, **304**, 294–296.

Britten N (1995). Patient demands for prescriptions in primary care. *British Medical Journal*, **310**, 1084–1085.

Britten N and Ukoumunne O (1997). The influence of patients' expectations of prescriptions on doctors' perceptions and the decision to prescribe. *British Medical Journal*, **315**, 1506–1510.

Buchanan A (1999). Independent inquiries into homicide. *British Medical Journal*, **318**, 1089–1090.

Bull JP (1959). The historical development of clinical therapeutic trials. *Journal of Chronic Diseases*, **10**, 218–248.

Chadwick D and Smith D (2002). The misdiagnosis of epilepsy. *British Medical Journal*, **324**, 495–496.

Cockburn J and Pit S (1997). Prescribing behaviour in clinical practice: patients' expectations and doctors' perceptions of patients' expectations – a questionnaire study. *British Medical Journal*, **315**, 520–523.

Cook RI, Render M and Woods DD (2000). Gaps in the continuity of care and progress on patient safety. *British Medical Journal*, **320**, 791–794.

Department of Health (2003). *Independent review of paediatric neurology services: Leicester.* Leicestershire, Northamptonshire and Rutland Strategic Health Authority.

Double D (2002). The limits of psychiatry. *British Medical Journal*, **324**, 900–904.

Even C, Siobud-Dorocant E and Dardennes RM (2000). Critical approach to antidepressant trials: Blindness protection is necessary, feasible and measurable. *British Journal of Psychiatry*, **177**, 47–51.

Gilley J (1994). Towards rational prescribing. *British Medical Journal*, **308**, 731–732.

Goldberg D and Huxley P (1992). *Common mental disorders.* London: Routledge.

Houston WR (1938). Doctor himself as therapeutic agent. *Annals of Internal Medicine*, **11**, 1416–1425.

Karlowski TR, Chalmers TC, Frenkel LD, *et al.* (1975). Ascorbic acid for the common cold. *Journal of the American Medical Association*, **231**, 1038–1042.

Kessler D, Bennewith O, Lewis G and Sharp D (2002). Detection of depression and anxiety in primary care: Follow up study. *British Medical Journal*, **325**, 1016–1017.

Kirsch I, Moore TJ, Scoboria A and Nicholls SS (2002). The emperor's new drugs: an analysis of antidepressant medication data submitted to the U.S. Food and Drug Administration. *Prevention and Treatment*, **5**, Article 23, posted July 15, 2002. Available at www.journals.apa.org/prevention/volume5/toc-ju115–02.html.

Linjakumpu T, Hartikainen S, Klaukka T, Veijola J, Kivela SL and Isoaho R (2002). Use of medications and polypharmacy are increasing among the elderly. *Journal of Clinical Epidemiology*, **55**, 809–817.

Little P, Everitt H, Williamson I, Warner G, Moore M, Gould C, Ferrier K and Payne S (2001). Preferences of patients for patient centred approach to consultation in primary care: observational study. *British Medical Journal*, **322**, 468–472.

Martin PJ, Young G, Enevoldson TP and Humphrey PR (1997). Overdiagnosis of TIA and minor stroke: experience at a regional neurovascular clinic. *Quarterly Journal of Medicine*, **90**, 759–763.

McIntyre N and Popper K (1983). The critical attitude in medicine: the need for a new ethics. *British Medical Journal*, **287**, 1919–1923.

Melander H, Ahlqvist-Rastad J, Meijer G and Beermann B (2003). Evidence b(i)ased medicine—selective reporting from studies sponsored by pharmaceutical industry: review of studies in new applications. *British Medical Journal*, **326**, 1171–1173.

Myers MG, Reeves RA, Oh PI and Joyner CD (1996). Overtreatment of hypertension in the community? *American Journal of Hypertension*, **9**, 419–425.

Nash H (1962). The double-blind procedure: Rationale and empirical evaluation. *Journal of Nervous and Mental Disease*, **134**, 24–47.

National Institute for Health Care Management (2002). *Prescription drug expenditures in 2001: Another year of escalating costs.* Washington: NIHCM.

Nimnuan C, Hotopf M and Wessely S (2000). Medically unexplained symptoms: How often and why are they missed? *Quarterly Journal of Medicine*, **93**, 21–28.

Nimnuan C, Hotopf M and Wessely S (2001). Medically unexplained symptoms: An epidemiological study in seven specialities. *Journal of Psychosomatic Research*, **51**, 361–367.

Perucca E (2002). Overtreatment in epilepsy: Adverse consequences and mechanisms. *Epilepsy Research*, **52**, 25–33.

Pillans PI and Roberts MS (1999). Overprescribng: have we made any progress? *Australian and New Zealand Journal of Medicine*, **29**, 485–486.

Porter R (2000). *Quacks. Fakers and charlatans in English medicine.* Stroud: Tempus.

Rosen MP, Sands DZ and Kuntz KM (2000). Physicians' attitudes towards misdiagnosis of pulmonary embolism: A utility analysis. *Academic Radiology*, **7**, 14–20.

Roth M and Kroll J (1986). *The reality of mental illness.* Cambridge: Cambridge University Press.

Royal College of Paediatrics and Child Health (2001). *Independent Performance Review of Dr. Andrew Holton, Leicester Royal Infirmary.* Available at http://www.uhl-tr.nhs.uk/news/epilepsy/full_report.pdf.

Shapiro AK and Shapiro E (1997). *The powerful placebo. From ancient priest to modern physician.* London: John Hopkins.

Skrabanek P and McCormick J (1998). *Follies and fallacies in medicine*, 3rd edn. Whithorn: Tarragon Press.

Stewart M, Brown JB, Weston WW, McWhinney IR, McWilliam CL and Freeman TR (2003). *Patient-centred medicine. Transforming the clinical method*, 2nd edn. Abingdon: Radcliffe Medical Press.

Tapp A, Wood AE, Secrest L, Erdmann J, Cubberley L and Kilzieh N (2003). Combination antipsychotic therapy in clinical practice. *Psychiatric Services*, **54**, 55–59.

Uldall P, Alving J, Buchholt J, Hansen L and Kibak M (2001). Evaluation of a tertiary referral epilepsy centre for children. *Presentation of the 4th International of the European Paediatric Neurology Society Meeting*, Baden-Baden, September 2001. Abstract 146. Available at http://www.akau.ch/epns 2001.

Walshe K and Higgins J (2002). The use and impact of inquiries in the NHS. *British Medical Journal*, **325**, 895–900.

Wheeldon NM, MacDonald TM, Flucker CJ, McKendrick AD, McDevitt DG and Struthers AD (1993). Echocardiagraphy in chronic heart failure in the community. *Quarterly Journal of Medicine*, **86**, 17–23.

Winters E, ed. (1951/2). *The collected papers of Adolf Meyer*, **vol. 1–4**. Baltimore: Johns Hopkins Press.

Young JH (1992). *The medical messiahs*. Princetown University Press.

Zubcevic S, Gavranovic M, Catibusic F and Buljina A (2001). Frequency of misdiagnosis of epilepsy in a group of 79 children with diagnosis of intractable epilepsy. Presentation at the 4th International longness of the European Paediatric Neurology Society meeting, Baden-Baden Abstract 337. Available at http://www.akw.ch/edns2001.

Index

Lightning Source UK Ltd.
Milton Keynes UK
UKHW020636190223
417171UK00003B/273